1984

Hospice U.S.A.

Hospice U.S.A.

**Austin H. Kutscher, Samuel C. Klagsbrun,
Richard J. Torpie, Robert DeBellis, Mahlon S. Hale
and Margot Tallmer, editors**

with the editorial assistance of
Lillian G. Kutscher

New York

Columbia University Press

1983

Columbia University Press
New York   Guildford, Surrey

Library of Congress Cataloging in Publication Data
Main entry under title:

Hospice U.S.A.

  (Foundation of Thanatology series)
  Bibliography: p.
  Includes index.
  1. Terminal care facilities—United States—Addresses,
essays, lectures. 2. Terminal care—Unites States—
Addresses, essays, lectures. 3. Terminal care—Moral
and ethical aspects—Addresses, essays, lectures.
I. Kutscher, Austin H. II. Title: Hospice USA.
III. Series: Foundation of Thanatology series
(Columbia University Press) [DNLM:. Hospices—United
States. WX 28.6 AAl H8]
R726.8.H674 1983   362.1'75   82-17705
ISBN 0-231-05082-8

Clothbound editions of Columbia University Press books
are Smyth-sewn and printed on permanent and durable
acid-free paper

Contents

Part III. Hospice Caregiving

Part IV. Helping the Dying: Caregiver Approaches

Part V. Patients and Illnesses

Preface

Austin H. Kutscher and Lillian G. Kutscher

It is relevant to pause in midstream to survey the past history and current status of the hospice movement in the United States and to speculate on its future. What of that which is now functioning will survive? How far beyond their beginnings and in what directions can currently developing hospice programs expand? As a philosophy of caregiving for the terminally ill, the hospice system has imposed limitations on the therapeutic interventions that should be provided for dying patients. Can we live with these limitations?

Even as an economic crusade against ever-increasing medical costs advances in the United States, and with it restrictions on renovating existing facilities or building replacement facilities, a humanistic crusade has been launched on behalf of an innovative modality of caregiving for a specific population of patients. For all our concern about humanitarian caregiving for dying patients and the members of their families, the bottom line of financial feasibility still looms, likely to be the determining factor behind whether an enlightened concept will be accorded recognition and a high priority on the list of what our society will try to accomplish. On the balance sheet, presumed cost effectiveness has been a most valuable ally of the hospice concept of patient care.

Congress has recognized hospice services as a benefit under Medicare, offering funding for hospice programs as an alternative to the cure-oriented system of traditional hospital care or the rather neutral care offered by nursing homes. Approaches to dying at home for those with a life expectancy of six months or less are the cornerstones of both cost containment and humanitarian efforts in this area. The Congressional Budget Office has estimated that about 50,000 persons are now being served to one degree or another by hospice programs annually; 95 percent are cancer patients and 60 percent of these are eligible for Medicare. The average length of stay in such a program has varied between 35 to 62 days, and increased savings have been projected when comparing the kind of care to be given in this manner with the kind of care offered in an acute care hospital. In its limited endorsement of the hospice concept of care, the health insurance industry is experimenting with reimbursement for services that would be provided by an existing home health or inpatient benefit plan that will mobilize community resources and augment existing services for the patient only when necessary. With the bias directed toward home care, the conclusion is often offered that the cost of caring for our terminally ill can be lowered substantially.

The supportive funding now forthcoming has been confined to demonstration programs and has a time limit. The stronger entities within the hospice framework are receiving help: a small number of free-standing buildings; home care programs organized within communities, some hospital-based and others community-agency based; and a very limited number of beds in acute care hospitals for patients who require sophisticated, personalized responses to relieve their physical pain and somatic complaints.

Where home care benefits are provided by a state, family members, with assistance from committed caregiving professionals and a cohort of trained volunteers, are attempting to avoid or postpone the institutionalization of a dying loved one and to offer what comfort they can within the sanctuary of the home. When this can be done, the holistic dimensions of hospice care can be maintained. Yet there are illnesses whose demands on caregiving time and family or third party money are beyond satisfying without calling upon institutional facilities. Perhaps circumstances such as these latter have almost mandated that the cancer patient be the model patient for a model kind of caregiving, for when we think of hospice care, we usually think in terms of the cancer patient, despite the needs of others stricken by equally stressful diseases.

So, at midstream, we review what has been initiated as an alternative form of care with an exalted philosophy and great promises for many terminally ill patients. Changes in existing medical care systems have been sought from a base in good conscience but have been brought to public attention and formal establishment through appeals to judicial and legislative bodies. This is evidenced in court decisions that have upheld the rights of patients and families to discontinue life-prolonging measures and in the "right to die" laws passed in many states. In the courts, what is just and right is not subjected to the rules of triage but to the inalienable rights of every citizen. Our constitutional structures take seriously the concept of protecting the individual from harm or undue suffering. Even with these safeguards, it is wise to question how, how long, and how well the hospice system—under many painful pressures—will survive with all of its ideals intact.

Professionals are needed within every system of the health industry. Although these providers are available, there are scarcely enough to meet the needs of both the acutely ill but curable and the chronically ill but incurable. The tragic aspects of triage on a national scale have never been exemplified better than in our struggle to establish hospice programs for the terminally ill. Institutions are available to provide many kinds of care, but there are not enough of these to fulfill every need of every patient and every family. Many parallels can be drawn between the plight of the dying and the plight of those who are mentally ill or severely retarded, particularly in relation to opportunities and obligations for caregiving in the home and in the community. No resources are limitless—not those of money, energy, commitment, professional expertise; and certainly not those of dedicated helping hands, either volunteer or paid. The largest single general issue facing our country is the allocation of resources. For all our expert planning, we seem to do this task poorly. How high a priority will the triage approach give to the needs of dying individuals? When hospice programs meet resistance from many quarters, we should not be surprised: every group with its own interests to champion asks, If I am not for me, who will be for me? Lacking strength as a political constituency, terminal patients can be left without their proper share of anything. Emulating the hospice philosophy practiced in Great Britain, we still must question whether what has worked there can be as functional or adequately functional in our own country, which differs from Great Britain in so many ways.

Assuming that the hospice philosophy offers us the most effective approach to relieving the suffering of those in intractable pain and the emotional stress imposed on their family members, can we afford anything less than one or another version of it for those in need today—or, with a glimpse into the statistics that mark 33 percent of our population as potential victims of cancer, for many of us tomorrow? The issues of *Hospice U.S.A.* are not those of "to be or not to be," but of which design to activate, where, when, and how. How unfeeling if it should come to pass otherwise. Much of what have become insults to human dignity within the walls of hospitals were originally introduced as therapeutic advances to protect and save patients' lives. But, as stresses on it mounted, the hospital system felt forced to employ these same advances to protect itself rather than for the primary benefit of the patient. With traditional hospitals failing to adapt to the needs of dying patients, it is no wonder that people look elsewhere for solutions to the problems that accompany life's inevitabilities.

Statistics in hospice care benefits, aside from costs, are going to remain "soft." After all, it is difficult to measure tears, smiles, and frowns. The future of the hospice-philosophy structure may be divided between two models, those run by cost-conscious administrators, with an infusion of hard-nosed researchers and health planners, and those run by saints. The former will be more interested in quantative issues and the latter in qualitative issues. It is most unfortunate that saints cannot be cloned, or trained.

We should not allow two systems, hospital and hospice-philosophy, competing for community space, professional time, and the dollars budgeted for human services, to be perpetuated as hostile to each other. We should avoid erecting edifices for their own sake or making compromises that will see idealistic principles stifled in profit-motivated warehouses that give the lowest common denominator of care. Our concern should be to practice the ideals of the hospice philosophy wherever we can, not to construct buildings. If we are challenged by the triage mentality that forces us to allocate resources where they will be most significant in terms of preserving human productivity, we should not allow this to be at the expense of the humanitarian sensibilities that are everyone's birthright. In an era when TV sets, computer games, automobiles, and the other equally costly symbols of a consumer society appear to be necessities of life, it is not too much to hope for entitlements that evolve from compassion and empathy.

Human dignity derives from inner strength of the mind and spirit. The dignified person projects an image of spiritual and intellectual integrity—wholeness and control of the self. Within the hospice system, this becomes a reciprocating process between caregivers and care recipients. What the caregivers can provide dying patients fosters the patients' sense of self-worth and their role in the community, even if that community has shrunk to include only family members. What dying patients can provide for caregivers is a sense of eliteness, a sense of playing an exceptional role in people's lives.

We feel that the contributors to the hospice movement offer multiple insights into another important aspect of the American Way of Life. A decade or two from now the most commonly asked question about hospices may be: Was all the effort and commitment worthwhile? We can only hope that the answer—then as now—will be Yes.

Acknowledgment

The editors wish to acknowledge the support and encouragement of the Foundation of Thanatology in the preparation of this volume. All royalties from the sale of this book are assigned to the Foundation of Thanatology, a tax exempt, not for profit, public scientific and educational foundation.

Thanatology, a new subspecialty of medicine, is involved in scientific and humanistic inquiries and the application of the knowledge derived therefrom to the subjects of the psychological aspects of dying; reactions to loss, death, and grief; and recovery from bereavement.

The Foundation of Thanatology is dedicated to advancing the cause of enlightened health care for the terminally ill patient and his family. The Foundation's orientation is a positive one based on the philosophy of fostering a more mature acceptance and understanding of death and the problems of grief and the more effective and humane management and treatment of the dying patient and his bereaved family members.

Part I

The Hospice Movement:
Past and Present

1

The Hospice:
Its Changes
Through Time

Virginia Montero Seplowin
and Egilde Seravalli

The etymology of the word *hospice*, with its Latin and Greek roots, expresses the ancient impulse of welcoming and bestowing gifts on guests, of *hospitia* from which the words *hostel, hotel,* and *hospital* are also derived (*Encyclopedia Britannica* 1968, 11: 745-46). In ancient Greece, travelers were under the protection of Zeus Xenios, and custom dictated that they were to be fed, clothed, and entertained with no questions asked until these hospitia duties were performed. An object could be broken in two or exchanged between host and guest to symbolize the promise of return services.

The rise of the city-state led to the appointment of a hospe or host in a foreign territory to protect outbound citizens. This person acted as a consul and was not paid although he received privileges. Thus, private hospitality became public (*Encyclopedia Britannica* 1910, 13: 80). Later in Rome, the hospe entertained at public expense. When the hospitia practice was extended from one city-state to another, the hospe provided lodging and amusement in return for payment. In Rome, too, the tie between hospe and guest became an inviolable contract blessed by Jupiter Hospitalis.

There was also a corresponding attitude toward the ailing. The concept of a place where people go to die originated during the eras in history when plagues decimated a population. As early as 1134 B.C., healing sanctuaries existed in Greece. The outpatient clinic probably had its beginning there (Cohen 1979: 13-21). The early Egyptians and Orientals, as well as Greeks and Romans, used their temples, where healing was practiced, as places of refuge for the sick. In the sixth century B.C., Buddha and his son established a remarkable network of medical centers in India. With the rise of Christianity and later Mohammedanism, many religious orders had new concern for the blind, the crippled, the leper, and those whose illnesses were often fatal.

The deterioration of the Roman Empire brought changes to many hospice activities and new forms to private and public hospitality. The hospe now required letters of introduction from the well connected; other travelers were forced to go to lower rated hospices that fell into two general categories, secular and religious. The first offered a range of entertainment, including orgies, often in disreputable and nefarious atmospheres (Bronowski 1973: 141). The second emphasized hospitality for the sick and the poor. These religious centers, established at important junctures along the Roman highways, had started with simple informality. Dormitories were later built adjacent to these monasteries, and churches and clerics were assigned to look after the guests. The gesture of hospitia concerned itself with healing only secondarily.

In 1096, the Crusades, motivated by religious fervor, gave the hospices a significant impetus. The religious hospe, now including knights, began to defend its guests. The Hospitalers, a military order, established numerous hospitals throughout Europe and Syria, the most famous being the Order of St. John of Jerusalem. The nuns connected with that Order also established the Hospice of St. Mary Magdalene for women, attesting to the fact that women have been active in hospice work throughout history.

As the Church waxed in political power, it became the means by which its adherents gained education, power, and prestige. Medicine came under its control. Practices were, however, inconsistent and tended to succumb to superstition. In addition, physicians, trained primarily as academicians with little knowledge of anatomy, read surgery instructions from ancient books while assistants actually performed the operations (Bronowski). The status of all medical services suffered. In an effort to impose controls, the Church issued an edict prohibiting monks and clerics from performing surgery. These events were part of a larger change taking place. Because the status of the hospe had so greatly declined, in 1473 the English petitioned that the professional name be changed to innkeeper (*Encyclopedia Britannica* 1968 11: 742-46).

What was going on to so thoroughly discredit hospitia? To understand the intruding forces, it is necessary to trace the history of plagues. Humanity had experienced pandemics since prehistoric times, but the first recorded plague took place among the Philistines. Samuel 5:6 states, "and he destroyed them and smote them with emerods." Samuel 6:19 adds "and he smote of the people fifty thousand three score and ten men: and the people lamented because the Lord had smitten many of them with a great slaughter" (American Bible Society edition 1875: 256-57). The first recorded pandemic plague took place between A.D. 540 and 558 in Byzantium during the reign of Justinian and was a factor in the destruction of the Empire (Oman 1897: 101-2). In the twelfth and thirteenth centuries, leprosy burst upon Europe (Cohen 1979: 19). Lazarettos, named after the Biblical leper Lazarus and the Order of St. Lazar, were hurriedly built. These crude structures on the edges of town or on offshore islands attempted to isolate the mysterious victims from the terrorized community; they were the only refuge available to the fatally ill. Their aim was to alleviate spiritual suffering because medical knowledge was still ignorant of the etiology of diseases. About 4,000 lazarettos existed in France and Germany and more than 200 in England and Scotland.

In the fourteenth century, the bubonic plague infected two-thirds of Europe and caused the death of 25 million people. In the process, it changed the course of history. Societies broke down; government, commerce, and the Church lost authority. The plague led to civil disobedience and agrarian revolts; indirectly, it brought about the Reformation. Mental aberrations and religious fanaticism further affected large masses of the population. It is now known that plagues cover vast areas and reemerge after centuries of quiescence. They not only drain and overwhelm community resources but also strike at the most basic group survival fears. History records that there is much rejection, revulsion, and shame connected with disease. In countering these attitudes, many outstanding religious men and women made their contribution to society.

The crisis that devastated Europe in the Middle Ages was simultaneously accompanied by a creative force. Beginning in the fourteenth century, the Renaissance spanned 300 years of vigorous humanistic and scientific explorations.

Alchemy introduced minerals to medicine. Syphilis, recognized as a separate disease by 1500, was treated with mercury. Although alchemy eventually fell into disrepute, its tools and methods were taken over in the sixteenth century by the new study of medical chemistry. Science once again guided medicine (Margenau et al. 1961: 90).

In northern Europe, the Renaissance coincided with the Reformation. Early in the sixteenth century, Henry VII of England spearheaded secular support to hospitals when he endowed St. Bartholomew's. Later in that same century, Henry VIII outlawed the monasteries and removed the direct influence of the Church on medicine. Together with the Closure Movement, which disenfranchised many, the shutdown of the monasteries created a huge outcast group. Death was common in open fields and on the streets. These conditions moved the citizens of London to petition Henry for lodging for the unfortunates. The petition was not granted, but it led to the humanitarian Poor Laws (Stoddard 1978: 61).

Hospitals had not always cared for the sick, but in the eighteenth century, the idea of founding charities to care for the poor sick took hold. The principles of private and public hospitals—now interpreted as charity—saw another change. Voluntary hospitals, as private hospitals were called, were augmented by workhouses that accommodated the poor and their families (Smith 1964: 2-4). Some form of work was assigned as a means of covering expenses. Admission was restricted and services were extended to the poor—not the destitute. In fact, hospitals, fearing the shame of pauper funerals and not wanting to underwrite the expense, often had the patients guarantee funeral costs before admission.

At the beginning of the nineteenth century, despite the growth of science, medical knowledge consisted of "nurse's gossip, sick men's fancies and the crude compilation of a blundering empiricism" (Smith

1964: 8). Little effective medicine existed, and what health care prevailed was better received at home. Effective home remedies, handed down from generation to generation, were thought to be more reliable than hospital treatment, which people dreaded. Physicians and medical directors now came from the elite classes, but they were better trained in the classics than in anatomy. Nurses were "little more than domestics of a rough and coarse type" and were treated as such (*ibid.*). It was a painful maturation period for medicine. Hospitals, which began as centers where physicians did charitable work, now became centers for teaching and research. The few physicians in the lucrative teaching positions did not want to give up or share them. The larger group of practitioners and the younger medical graduates were forced to open new fields. Specialized hospitals were organized with mixed motivations: concern for new knowledge and personal status (*ibid.*, p. 19). Buttressed by the philosophy of enlightenment and a growing belief in the intellect, medical practitioners saw the patient more and more as an object. In 1863, Florence Nightingale wrote, "The very first requirement of a hospital [is] that it should do the sick no harm" (*ibid.*, p. 1).

It was a co-worker of Nightingale's, Sister Mary Aikenhead of the Irish Sisters of Charity, who opened a hospice in Dublin in the late nineteenth century (Stoddard 1978: 87). Little is known about her, but it is certain that Sister Mary spent time in the Vincent de Paul hospices in France. Numerous other hospices existed in England by the end of the nineteenth century, but the one most like the Irish hospice was St. Joseph's Hospice, founded by the English Sisters of Charity in 1906. It was here during the 1950s and 1960s that Dr. Cicely Saunders developed her work in the control of pain and then went on to establish St. Christopher's Hospice in 1967.

A stream of concerned professionals from the United States has visited and continues to visit St. Christopher's to study it as a model for the caregiving of the terminally ill. The hospice movement has crossed the Atlantic to the United States. Beginning with the hospice that pioneered in 1974 as the first hospice service in the United States in New Haven, Connecticut (now called the Connecticut Hospice), the movement grew until, by 1979, the National Hospice Organization listed 209 hospices incorporated in the United States (Cohen 1979: 208-34).

Derived from an ancient value, present-day hospice means an attitude, a concept, a service. As a service, it may take place in an institution exclusively devoted to it or may be practiced in alternative sites. It may be part of a hospital service, in a separate unit, or as an interdisciplinary program covering terminally ill patients assigned to rooms throughout the building. It may include a home care program providing round-the-clock team service or an outpatient or day care program, or it may be sponsored by one institution or in cooperation with others. Whatever its form, the ultimate goal is the same: to respect the dying and allow them to end their days in harmony.

Since the new hospice practices have been reclaimed from ancient and medieval concepts of compassion, caring, and concern, it is suggested that another term, with an analogous history of time and place, be used in connection with hospice. The term is *pietas*, an ancient Greek word for devotion to the gods, denoting giving from the richness and fullness of oneself to someone in need. Hospice and pietas link the philosophic and practical attitudes that the sick and life-threatened need from society.

References

Bronowski, J. 1973. *The Ascent of Man*. Boston, Massachusetts: Little, Brown and Co.

Cohen, K. P. 1979. *Hospice*. Germantown, Maryland: Aspen Systems Corp.

The Holy Bible. 1875. New York: American Bible Society.

"Hospice." 1910. *Encyclopedia Britannica*, Vol. 13.

"Hospice." 1968. *Encyclopedia Britannica*, Vol. 11.

"Hotel." 1968. *Encyclopedia Britannica*, Vol. 11.

Margenau, J. et al. 1961. *The Scientist*. New York: Time Inc.

Oman, W. C. 1897. *The Byzantine Empire*. New York: G. P. Putnam's Sons.

Smith, B. A. 1964. *The Hospitals of England and Wales, 1800–1948*. Cambridge, Massachusetts: Harvard University Press.

Stoddard, S. 1978. *The Hospice Movement*. Briarcliff Manor, New York: Stein and Day.

2

The Hospice Movement
and the Acceptance of Death

John E. Hare

There are dangers whenever a revolutionary idea leaves the stage of initial formulation and implementation and becomes the basis of a widespread movement. The hospice idea is now going through this transition.[1] The dangers can be seen by an examination of the nursing home movement, which began bravely but became so successful that nursing homes are now part of the established fabric of our society. In this case, the penalty of success has been that the ideal has been diluted and in some places abused. One of the dangers facing the hospice movement is that the original idea, which was one of great flexibility, may become too rigid. Clearly a tension exists here between the desire to stay as close as possible to the original idea and the desire to allow that idea to be applied in varying ways as it is appropriate to various differing contexts. An analogy may be drawn with the endless battles within the Christian Church about how far a local group can diverge from the interpretation of the faith accepted by the ecclesiastical hierarchy without being declared heretical.

Many issues are involved in the variegation of the original idea of a hospice. Should all types of terminal illness be accepted, or may admission be restricted to cancer patients? Should continued chemotherapy and radiation therapy be allowed for hospice patients? Should hospices always be in free-standing buildings, or may they also be part of larger hospitals? Are hospice patients permitted to request single rooms if they are, for example, grossly disfigured by disease or surgery? It is not hard to think of a number of similar issues.

The question, in Aristotelian terms, is what is essential to a hospice and what is merely accidental. There is probably a continuum here, with clear cases at either end. Not all hospices have beautiful gardens like those at St. Christopher's in London. But all hospices *do* have to emphasize palliation and the care of the whole family. Between these is a large area of uncertainty and a corresponding danger that whoever establishes standards may draw the line too narrowly.

An added twist to the difficulty is that the original idea included an unusual degree of openendedness. Cicely Saunders says, "You are asked to forget one special place and to put the patients we discuss into your own setting, translating general principles into particular situations."[2] Thus a paradoxical choice arises between accepting the original blueprint without the openendedness or accepting the openendedness and changing some details of the blueprint. This is apparently paradoxical because those details are no more original than the flexible attitude that finds them inessential.

One might argue that it does not matter whether the label "hospice" is attached to an institution or not. But the situation is complicated because the label is itself significant in attracting support, both financial and political. It does matter, therefore, whether or not the decision is that the label may be used.

One particular form of potentially dangerous rigidification is the simplistic application of Kübler-Ross' five stages, which are becoming a form of orthodoxy in the hospital context. This tendency needs to be resisted. Kübler-Ross' work has had tremendous value in bringing into the public eye the question of how patients with a terminal illness should be treated. She has also been consistently supportive of the hospice movement.[3] But there is an interpretation of her work that holds that the five stages—denial, anger, bargaining, depression, and acceptance— *ought* to follow each other in the stated order and that if the patient does not reach acceptance by the time of death, there is something wrong either with the patient or the hospital staff.

I have argued that Kübler-Ross does not herself say that the stages have to come in any particular order, although she does say that acceptance should come at the end.[4] It was also suggested that the term *acceptance* itself can bear many different interpretations. Three attitudes were singled out and called "Stoic," "Christian," and "Humanist." The Stoic attitude is that death itself (not just the dying process) is a natural part of life just like birth and that it is part of the providential. It is a friend and not an enemy, and to fear it is to fail to live in accordance with nature and to reach the chief human good. The attitude that was called Christian is that death is not a friend but rather "the last enemy," with an intimate connection to sin. Death is not to be feared, because the enemy has been defeated, not because he is not an enemy. In this view, death is not part of God's original plan for humanity but is now for almost all human beings a necessary step toward seeing Him face to face.

The third attitude, labeled Humanist, is that death is in fact the end of one's existence. As Heidegger would say, "Human Being is Being unto Death."[5] There is no need to focus attention on this. But it is possible rather to concentrate on settling one's affairs with one's family and living each moment of dying to the full. To see death this way is to refuse to blur the recognition that it is a necessary and final evil and to refuse also to let this recognition dominate the end of life.

These attitudes are described only briefly here, for there are likely to be as many attitudes toward death as there are people. Moreover, the views so labeled—Stoic, Christian, and Humanist—have often been merged so that there can be found Christian Stoics, Stoic Humanists, and Humanist Christians. It is useful to try to isolate these three components for the sake of clarity; it is particularly useful in reference to a discussion of Kübler-Ross since she seems to take a fairly pure form of the Stoic view.

It is, perhaps, misleading to call her view Stoic, for she is not likely to have come across it in this form. More likely is that she met the view in some form of Eastern wisdom. Well-known and intriguing parallels exist between some Stoic views and, for example, the Bhagavad Gita, even though there is no reliable evidence of historical contact in either direction. J. Bruce Long wrote a summary of Hindu and Buddhist attitudes to death, "The Death That Ends Death in Hinduism and Buddhism," which was included in Kübler-Ross' *Death: The Final Stage of Growth* (1975). Long sums up both Eastern traditions by saying, "That person is freed from the fetters of death and all its attendant anxieties, who meets death as a companion to life, in the spirit of rational and tranquil acceptance."

Kübler-Ross is herself committed to a belief in reincarnation. But there are other parallels that are relevant to a discussion of death and dying. The Gita stresses that to be freed from the sway of death, it is necessary to reach a state of desirelessness in which pain and pleasure, gain and loss, victory and defeat are equally little regarded.[6] The Stoics called these pairs and others like them "the indifferents." For them the only thing to be desired was virtue; with respect to everything else, they recommended *apatheia*—an absence of emotional attachment.[7] Kübler-Ross would urge us to escape "the illusory urgencies of the immediate."[8] What is immortal or eternal for her is the soul or spirit.

In Buddhist terms, the Self that perishes with the body is not the True Self. The distinction has often been drawn between a belief in the immortality of the soul (which is often found together with a belief in reincarnation) and a belief in resurrection. What is realized by someone who is released from the cycle of birth and death is that "the boundless light of this true Reality is yourself, your own true self."[9] The Stoics would say that the wisdom that is in the sage is the wisdom of the cosmos. Kübler-Ross would say that "there is a source of goodness, light, and strength greater than any of us individually, yet still within us all," and that "each essential self has an existence that transcends the finiteness of the physical and contributes that greater power."[10]

The purpose of this paper is not to explore all the similarities and differences among Stoicism, Hinduism, Buddhism, and the work of Kübler-Ross. Suffice it to suggest that there are some parallels. Nor is my purpose to argue the merits of this group of views. Kübler-Ross' out-of-the-body experiences have been seized by the media for their news value and are not relevant to this discussion. That any of this development was necessarily implicit in her first book is not clear. But she has continued to explore her own understanding of what "acceptance" means. Indeed, she apparently claims to have felt herself to have reached a permanent state of acceptance.[11] When she talks about acceptance now, there is inevitably a more specific content to the term, and this *is* relevant to our present topic.

The content Kübler-Ross gives to acceptance would not matter so much if her account were purely descriptive—if she were merely describing the stages through which she has observed her patients move. But it has become increasingly clear that while she believes that the other four stages may come in any order and some of them may not come at all, she believes it desirable that the stage of acceptance come last. This claim is normative or prescriptive and not merely descriptive. Thus, Hans Mauksch talks about "the privilege of helping the human being who is dying to work through to the stage of acceptance."[12] Mwalimu Imara says: "Going through the five stages of the terminal person's grief is a process moving toward a blessing, 'acceptance.'" He talks also about a research project undertaken to gain understanding of "the religious dynamics behind the denial process and the terminally ill patient's resistance to moving through to acceptance."[13] If acceptance is seen as normative, as the goal of care, then it becomes extremely important to determine what the conceptual framework is behind its prescription.

My thesis here is that there are many possible frameworks in which acceptance could find a place. Three of these were identified above. What is dangerous to assume is that most patients will have established their lives within any one of these.

Kübler-Ross is especially vulnerable to this danger because she wants to insist that "all people are basically alike; they all share the same fears and the same grief when death occurs"; and she cherishes the hope that "in the decades to come we may see one universe, one humankind, one religion that unites us all in a peaceful world."[14] This is not an unreasonable hope if we can suppose that there is already a religion that can be seen underneath all the differing dogmas and creeds of the world's present faiths and can be believed more fundamental than any of them. This seems to be the view of Imara in the final essay of her volume; his theological stance is at many points close to that of Paul Tillich. Tillich is quoted as describing the experience of being blessed, or the experience of grace, as follows: "And nothing is demanded of this experience, no religious or moral or intellectual presupposition, nothing but acceptance." Imara himself states that "*how* we interact with one another and *how* we experience ourselves are more important for dying persons than the content of their religious myths."[15]

If, however, there is not a fundamental religion already shared by all humankind, or at least by all those who are dying, it becomes important to allow patients to move, if they want to move at all, toward a kind of acceptance that is consistent with their *own* conceptual frameworks.[16] What makes it harder for the staff to be as openminded as this is that each of the three attitudes toward death—the Stoic, the Christian, and the Humanist—is likely to call the other two a form of denial. From a Stoic point of view, acceptance means more than emotional adjustment to the fact of death. "Emotional adjustment includes the concept of inner peace and self-possession, but it is not the same as ... acceptance."[17] In this view, a patient may find satisfactory meaning in the face of pain, helplessness, changing relationships, separations, and losses. He may even find a satisfactory answer to the question "Of what value am I now?" and still not have reached acceptance. What more would be required? It seems the patient has not accepted that it is only the body that dies; or perhaps he has not been released from the attachments to the desires of day-to-day living. But this means that to the Stoic the Humanist is still in a stage of denial because he does not believe in an afterlife or even in the beneficial effects of his present life spreading from generation to generation as long as the human race survives. He may be totally absorbed in the day-to-day running of his few remaining days, and he may choose not to think about his rapidly approaching death. From the Humanist point of view, this might be called acceptance. But for the Stoic it is likely to be called denial. The reverse is also the case. The Humanist will no doubt interpret the Stoic as one desperately trying to blur the reality of extinction by entertaining myths about survival, cosmic wisdom, or boundless light.

Acceptance in this context is an evaluative and not a purely descriptive term. The phrase "the acceptance of death" would be purely descriptive if it referred to the mere assent to the proposition "I am going to die." But as the phrase is usually used in the literature of thanatology, it refers to this assent and to a proper attitude toward approaching death. But what is called a proper attitude depends on the conceptual framework of the person evaluating it. A person who holds one of the three attitudes distinguished above will be likely to disagree with the attitudes of people who hold one of the other two, and will therefore not categorize them as having reached the stage of acceptance. There is a correlative point about the phrase "the denial of death." As this is usually used within thanatology, it refers, not merely to the refusal to assent to the proposition "I am going to die," but also to the refusal to adopt a "healthy" attitude to one's approaching death. Acceptance and denial are thus both evaluative terms in this context, and this is why the same person can be said in one value framework to be accepting and in another to be denying.

If the point is correct, it is an injustice to a patient to try to move him through to a stage defined in terms of a framework he does not believe in. One of the strengths of the original hospice concept was that it did not recommend this. Cicely Saunders said that "a patient needs the chance to handle his experiences in a way that will make them significant or at least bearable to him, and it is he who should decide how he will do this." [18] All the hospice people I have talked to have said that if a patient wants to deny his approaching death, and to continue doing so until he dies, that is fine. This does not show that there is something wrong with the patient or the staff. Some of them have also said, from experience with patients, that acceptance is a happier stage to be in. But this is quite consistent, for it does not imply that the patient should be helped or moved in this direction. It *would* imply this except for the recognition that the process of trying to move the patient from one stage to another is likely to do more harm than good, given the probabilities of his reaching acceptance.

Because of the evaluative character of the term, it is extremely difficult to say how many people reach acceptance, but the probability of reaching the full stage as described by Kübler-Ross may be rather low. In any case, the patient is at his most vulnerable in the terminal period. He needs all the scanty defenses he can muster from his past against pain, isolation, and the imminence of the unknown. To suggest even implicitly that his basic value framework is deficient is to shake those defenses and thus do him a great injury.

Those who want to work in a hospice setting, volunteers for example, are carefully screened to exclude those who are too eager to share their religious views with the patients. This is not to say that the staff are not usually religious people. The reverse is the case. In my own limited experience, hospice workers are usually those people who do not impose on others and who are acutely sensitive to the need to respect whatever beliefs about himself and the world a patient may have come in with. To cite Saunders once more: "We cannot impose our own beliefs upon [the patient], but if we believe that there is a meaning, our silent steadiness will help him to find his own way through."[19]

There is a danger that Kübler-Ross' five stages may be simplistically applied so that the staff try to move the patients through them and give a content to the stage of acceptance that derives from a particular conceptual framework or family of views. It would be a shame if it became a party line, so to speak, in the hospice movement, either that pressure of any kind should be put on patients to reach acceptance or that any one definition of acceptance should be adopted. For both of these developments would be at variance with the original concept and would make the movement itself less suitable to a highly pluralist society.

If the goal is, as it is so often said to be, to learn from the patient, we are hindering this learning to the extent that we prescribe in advance what sort of acceptance we are going to be looking for. It is surely better to restrict the term *acceptance* to a purely descriptive sense—namely, the assent to the proposition "I am going to die"—and to leave it to the patient to determine on the basis of his own life what attitude or conceptual framework this implies.

Notes

1. See *The Hospice Movement* by S. Stoddard (Briarcliff, New York: Stein and Day, 1978).

2. *Contact*, Supplement 38, Summer 1972, pp. 12-18. In her introduction to Richard Lamerton's book, *Care of the Dying* (Hove, England: Priory Press, 1973), Dr. Saunders says, "Because he is an enthusiast who gives us a number of dogmatic statements, Dr. Lamerton stimulates us to test and try for ourselves." If she has made any dogmatic statements of her own, she would no doubt want us to treat them in the same way.

3. Especially in *To Live Until We Say Goodbye* (Englewood Cliffs, New Jersey: Prentice-Hall, 1978) and *Death: The Final Stage of Growth* (Englewood Cliffs, New Jersey: Prentice-Hall, 1975).

4. J. E. Hare, "Denial of Death," in S. G. Wolf et al., eds., *Caregiving in the Community Hospital: For the Terminally Ill and the Bereaved* (New York: Arno Press/A New York Times Company, 1981).

5. Martin Heidegger, *Being and Time* (New York: Harper and Row, 1962).

6. *Bhagavad Gita*, ii 70, 71; and v 28.

7. See F. H. Sandbach, *The Stoics* (London: Norton, 1975), chapter 3.

8. *Death: The Final Stage of Growth*, p. 167.

9. *Ibid.*, p. 69.

10. *Ibid.*, p. 166.

11. Ann Nietzke, "The Miracle of Kübler-Ross," *Human Behavior*, 1977; reprinted in *Cosmopolitan*, February 1980, p. 306.

12. *Death: The Final Stage of Growth*, p. 12.

13. *Ibid.*, p. 154.

14. *Ibid.*, pp. 2-3.

15. *Ibid.*, p. 154.

16. See James C. Carpenter, "Accepting Death: A Critique of Kübler-Ross," Hastings Center Report, October 1979.

17. Raymond G. Carey, "Living Until Death: A Program of Service and Research for the Terminally Ill," in *Death: The Final Stage of Growth*, pp. 77-81.

18. *District Nursing* (now *Queens Nursing Journal*), September 1965, pp. 149-150, 154.

19. *Ibid.*

3

The Hospice Community as Reform

Henry J. Wald

There are internal and external forces that ultimately shape evolving institutions within the American health system. In roughly the last two decades, the reform called the "hospice movement" has evolved in the United States and, in general, has been composed, either in total or in segments, of home care services, changes in hospital programs, and often, new autonomous institutions. Its character, shaped by vision, values, and new skills introduced by a very few leaders, has evolved into a reform. Like any reform, the hospice movement needs time and experience to formulate principles and enable the professionals to develop knowledge and expertise. Before integration into an established health care system, hospice needs a solid base, and that base requires time to gather facts, make tests, consider plans, and develop a sense of community within each setting. Now that reform movement in the United States has reached a critical stage. Largely through its extremely rapid expansion after 1975 when there were only three institutions giving care, there were, within the following three years, 78 institutions known to be giving care, and 213 others were planning services. In

October 1978, more than 1,000 people attended a meeting of the National Hospice Organization in Washington, D.C.

This satisfying reform is also a cause for corresponding alarm, for it distracts practitioners from their original goals because of the involvement of other groups—professional health care people, consumers, journalists, entrepreneurs, political strategists, management consultants, fund raisers, and so forth.

Another force acting on the reform is the inertia of existing insitutions that is reflected in problems such as government licensing, finding public and private monies, operational funds, and so forth. Another diversion is the necessity to develop internal organization and functional relationships with other institutions in the total system. How this reform is integrated within the system will determine not only its ultimate scope but also its quality and longevity.

Max Weber, the German sociologist, recognized that every reform begins with dissatisfaction with an existing system and then develops ideas for a new approach. If ideas are to be kept alive, there must be mutual attention between the nourishing idealists and the policymakers (Weber 1964).

Cicely Saunders, Elizabeth Kübler-Ross, and Herman Feifel are among the people who have appeared on many public platforms. They have been influential over a 20-year period, and most particularly during the past 10 years insofar as hospice is concerned. What was absolutely unacceptable around 1958 became possible in 1960. The full impact of Dr. Saunders' theories and possibilities for adoption became apparent on her third visit to Yale in 1966, when she conducted a workshop. Then, five years later, an interdisciplinary group at Yale, under Dr. Saunders' inspiration, concluded that a hospice was needed in the greater New Haven area, a community of more than half a million people.

What we were facing then in New Haven must be considered in context as a high-risk involvement appropriate to the area and not necessarily applicable to other communities. Since that period, four other basic forms of hospice care have evolved. One is the home care hospice program. An example of this is the Hospice of Marin in California, although its staff also provides care for patients in several hospitals in the region.

There are also hospice teams in hospitals. One of the most prominent examples in New York City is St. Luke's Hospital Center, where an interdisciplinary hospice team works with the patients. There are palliative care units in hospitals. Dr. Balfour Mount's unit at the Royal Victoria Hospital in Montreal is separate from yet within the hospital and has an interdisciplinary approach and a home care team. There are also hospices with hospital affiliations and completely autonomous hospices. Each community has to determine its own needs, resources, goals, and objectives in forming new services or in reforming existing ones.

The decision-making process in New Haven led to an autonomous system and a physical facility because of the probability of success in an open system's working within existing institutions such as Yale-New Haven Medical Center (in contrast to a low probability of success within existing nursing home systems, which were in very bad condition at the time).

There are other crucial steps in development. The International Work Group on Death, Dying, and Bereavement, which meets every 18 months, had a group of thirty social scientists and caregivers who formulated assumptions and principles of caregiving in terminal illness (1979). That group advocates diversity in care as long as these basic principles are observed. Patients need an open system for care and also cure. These complementary approaches frequently overlap. There must be interchange so that the patient is assured of appropriate treatment throughout the illness. Communications and a working relationship between the idealists and the policymakers are necessary to keep the reform viable. That is a crucial point in the hospice movement in the United States. Inherent in all these reforms is an adversary position with regard to existing systems. Reformers are faced with the reactions their ideals cause on institutions with a vested interest in the status quo. The open system challenges multiple health agencies that operate separately.

The decision making in planning inevitably involves compromises; everyone involved must ask at each stage of development if the compromise is necessary and if the ideals can survive. Time is involved. St. Christopher's Hospice took twenty years after Dr. Saunders' first visions to open its doors. In the United States, the time has been between one and eight years for planning alone. The hospice started in New Haven in 1971. It met its first difficulties applying for state approval on the

Certificate of Need application. Connecticut's Commissioner on Hospitals and Health Care looked for a basis of comparison and struggled to identify the category of health-related institutions into which the hospice would fit for licensing. If it wasn't a hospital or a nursing home, what was it? What did it resemble most in the public health code? How could it be reimbursed in the existing system? Was legislation needed? Should hospices become a new and separate category of health institution? The commission was also concerned with capital and operative costs. The New Haven group, seeing the physical environment as a necessary component of therapy, faced the problem of explaining the significance of measuring the value of a therapeutic environment.

As the private process evolved, the New Haven Hospice was careful to select an architect who could adapt plans to the patient's life-style, allow family participation, and create an atmosphere where opportunity could grow. We had an unusual architect selection committee consisting of nurses, clergy, and a teenage survivor of a mother who had died during care in an exploratory study. There was agreement in the committee that they had particularly selected an architect who had considerable humility about the problem. He had no fixed ideas and was prepared to work with us in developing an innovative program.

Our architect, Lo Yi Chan, told us soon after his engagement that he felt the assignment involved a highly stressful series of problems for him. He thought it was necessary to first visit St. Christopher's, spend as much time as he could afford there (it turned out to be more than a week), and take along another person—his wife—who would be influenced by the stresses he anticipated and help him during design.

Later on, Mr. Chan was invited to speak before one of the open house programs that the Hospice Incorporated had for the community. He had done no design and was familiar only with the generalized program we had presented to all the architects being considered. Mr. Chan went through a carousel of 70 or 80 slides as fast as he could and said that these slides would illustrate what he then knew about hospice as a program. Frequently, clients, particularly those for whom he was designing residences, asked him, "What is the building going to look like?" He would say that he could not tell until he found out more about the family's way of life, habits, and family relationships. He saw the same thing with hospice, a need for a strong relationship between the patient and the rest of the world from which he is separated. "What does this mean to an architect? One thing it means to me is windows—open windows."

Then he showed us slides that were architectural statements of windows in igloos, office buildings, internal, external—and of what a patient sees lying down. Halfway through his presentation he had completely involved his audience, and we knew we had chosen the right architect.

The crucial issue is that each community must work to develop programs before it jumps into such aspects as physical settings. It must develop what it needs and deems most appropriate for its own community. From there on, the community must consciously create a somewhat ambiguous program so that the professional who is translating the program into the physical can have the greatest freedom within the design.

Acknowledgment

The author acknowledges the collaborative efforts of Florence S. Wald, R.N., M.S., and Zelda Foster, M.S.W., in the preparation of this report.

References

International Work Group in Death, Dying, and Bereavement. 1979. "Assumptions and Principles Underlying Standards for Terminal Care." *American Journal of Nursing* (February) 79:297-98.

Weber, M. 1964. *Theory of Social and Economic Organization,* trans. by T. Parsons, New York: The Free Press.

4

The Politics of Expanding Hospice Care

Samuel C. Klagsbrun

The exposure of the American public to the concept of the hospice through lectures, workshops, seminars, and community meetings is astonishingly great when compared with the actual number of patients and their families being cared for in this country within the framework of a realistic hospice philosophy. That there is deception relates to the fact that there are extremely few hospice beds available and few ongoing hospice home care services. Although many are learning about hospice concepts (and this, in itself, is beneficial for those patients being cared for by the informed caregiver), there is very little true practice of hospice concepts. Knowing that medication on schedule is not a proper approach to a patient in pain is a piece of knowledge derived from hospice experiences. Any nurse or physician can offer pain relief to patients by changing from the traditional to the hospice approach to pain management. This change is not, however, the same as the totally encompassing care system that is hospice.

Hospice care means family care. It means focusing on patients' needs, and these are clearly defined needs. It means preparation, pain management, and spiritual care. Such care can be made available not only to dying patients but also to all patients with any illness.

According to the idealistic definition of hospice care, there is only rare application of this particular kind of care in this country. Visiting nurse services have for some time been a major instrument in bringing good care to homebound patients. They have learned from the hospice approach and have practiced it. Some physicians have begun to pay attention to hospice care concepts and techniques. Exploratory ad hoc committees in major hospitals across the country are studying whether or not hospice care can be instituted as a "scatter bed" system in acute care hospitals or as a separate geographic boundary, usually in a teaching hospital. Certain community hospitals (e.g., Riverside Hospice in Boonton, New Jersey) have committed themselves to establishing a truly operative hospice. When that hospice was developed, major momentum came from the lay leadership in that town and not from medical professionals. The lay leaders pressed the staff to agree in principle to the establishment of a hospice. It was then left to the laypersons to develop plans to raise money and hire staff for the hospice, which has been located one mile down the road from the hospital. Many of the hospice's referrals come from those outside the official hospital family. Although the hospital staff has not been against the hospice, energy and control have come from other sources.

In New York City, the actual existence of a large hospice program still goes begging. A small but unique program has been introduced into St. Luke's Hospital, and progress in Connecticut is exemplified by the difficulties the New Haven Hospice had to endure before finally finding a site to build on and funds to finance construction. Another hospice in Arizona is in deep trouble, and one in California has functioned as a home care system with the aid of volunteers.

The number of services in this country that offer consultation and volunteer efforts to existing facilities exceeds the total number of beds that actually provide total hospice care. The actual number of beds occupied by dying patients in existing institutions with the label of "hospice" probably does not exceed 1,000.

Yet we have produced a national hospice organization, and the number of councils and committees, organizations, and community-based hospice groups is probably high. But how many full-time people expending energies in research, service, and administration are spending their time on actual hospice care? We have much more talk and organization apparatus than we have total comprehensive actual hospice care of the dying.

Is the lack of third-party support or the lack of substantial government assistance hampering us? Is it really true that others are at fault? The hospice service that exists in my hospital (Four Winds Hospital, Katonah, New York) exists simply because it was needed, without attention paid to outside intervention or support. Although it is small, it is real.

Patients and families need hospice care. The government does not want to hear about it, because it will inflate the budget. Insurance companies are too insecure to realize the financial benefits of any experimental program until someone else does it first and demonstrates that it is effective and, perhaps, profitable. Organized medical institutions will probably pay only lip service to hospice care. The work to be done cannot be done in newspapers or magazine articles, although these may prick some consciences. The work to be done is at the bedside of the dying patient.

Hospice work is lonely, hard, and frightening. It does not always engender gratefulness, and it frequently causes depression for everyone concerned. This work cannot be done alone; it is complicated. A community-based hospice that offers consultative help to families, physicians, or nurses must have actual hospital beds built into the system. These beds must be available at will to function as part of the hospice or to function in a hospice light. Hospice work therefore requires a cooperative effort that includes total care from hospital to home. Not every hospice patient will spend time in the hospital bed, but that bed must be ready if the patient needs it.

A hospice needs a chaplain, a social worker, physicians, nurses, an administrator, volunteers, and a psychiatrist who is knowledgeable in this area. A group of people who can take care of each other while they are taking care of dying patients and their families is needed. And with this community of people, a financial base is needed.

About 30 years ago, the focus was on the incidence of suicide in the United States. Suicide prevention centers were funded and established as a result of sound research into the problem and how to deal with it. At one time it seemed as if every town had a suicide hotline manned by volunteers. A current study of these original centers has been done and the original telephone numbers listed for them were called. There was hardly a single response. Most of those numbers still existed as expressions of a community's wishes, but there was no one manning the phones. Without a strong commitment by a community, no center will be effective or continue to exist. Even when the telephone listings were first published, most of the centers were taken care of by answering services. If a suicidal person were to call, the operator would say, "Just a minute. Give me your name and number and I'll have a doctor or someone call you back."

This same phenomenon should not occur in the hospice movement. A population in need of a hospice cannot hold onto the phone until someone decides to offer a helping hand. The answer is a hard-nosed consolidation—a tightening of criteria and a much more efficient way of focusing on the setting up of a small number of true hospices in this country in different locations and possibly with different aims to find out what is required to establish a hospice and who is going to foot the bill. If we cannot manage to do this, it will be apparent that we really do not care very much about old or dying people. Hospice care and the politics of hospice are entirely different. We have already spent too much time on the politics of hospice. It is now time to approach the real work of hospice—caring for the dying.

5

The Hospice Movement:
A Management Perspective

Joseph R. Proulx and Elizabeth J. Colerick

The hospice movement is an ideology that advocates holistic or "total" care of the dying person by addressing four pains: physical, emotional, social, and spiritual. In effect, hospice is a humane and caring approach to a meaningful death that begins where technology ends. The first hospice appeared in this country in 1974, and it is estimated that 200 such programs are presently offering care or are in the developmental stages. Observably, the need for hospice has stimulated a sweeping response in our society that, in turn, has produced action on the part of thousands. This goal-directed activity is truly the thrust of the hospice movement.

To date, most of the hospice literature speaks of isolated concepts such as death and dying; physical, psychological, social, and spiritual pain; and grief, loss, and family bereavement. Hospice encompasses, however, more than these subjective manifestations. From an institutional perspective, it is a major new service. When assuming this particular stance, the literature addresses an array of different and isolated topics such as funding, architecture and physical design, medication, palliative treatment, utilization of volunteers, and staff development programs.

What is crucial now is the need to embrace another view of hospice, one that delineates concrete administrative principles and managerial strategies to allow such a service to be carefully planned, effectively organized, skillfully led, and objectively evaluated. Both the hospice movement and its future development need a broad conceptual analysis firmly rooted in sound managerial elements of planning (P), organizing (O), leading (L), and evaluating (E). Theoretically, POLE is a symbol that represents the "process of management" (Kazmier 1974: 34-46; Stoner 1978: 17-20).

Because it is well recognized that a universal need for hospice exists, it seems appropriate to propose a practical universal model to guide the managers, leaders, and professionals who are attempting to bring this concept to fruition. POLE is adjustable to any program, system, or institution, regardless of size or mission. "Thus, whether in a small business firm, a governmental agency ·or a large corporation...whether on the general management level or in a specialized area of work, all managers are involved in carrying out the functions of planning, organizing, directing and controlling," (Kazmier, p. 35). The paradigm POLE outlines a pragmatic approach to hospice management that is simple, yet not simplistic. Its principles of planning, organizing, leading, and evaluating have the intrinsic ability to concretize the hospice concept.

In theory, the acronym POLE is symbolic. The components of POLE, although representations of the real world, must be empirically tested and explained. Through a semistructured interview with Susan Silver, the executive director of The Washington Hospice Society, theory melded into actual practice. Our purpose is to propose a general theoretical model that emphasizes managerial principles rather than clinical concepts for the analysis of any developing hospice. The interview is reproduced within the following four segments of the model.

Planning

In each component of the POLE paradigm, key statements or questions set the stage for further conceptual development. Thus, in planning, queries that must be addressed concern "what is to be done, when is it to be done, how is it to be done, and who is to do it?" (Steiner 1969: 7). Interestingly enough, the question "why" is frequently neglected in the management literature, and this is essential to answer because it defines the organization's *raison d'être*.

The planning function is critical to organizational effectiveness and efficiency. Planning focuses on organizational goals and addresses specific purposes and activities. Furthermore, it provides reference points to measure progress and to guide future action. As one author has so aptly stated, "planning provides the score from which the orchestra of the organization plays in harmony." (Stoner 1978: 92).

When the executive director of The Washington Hospice Society reviewed the planning function of her organization, she began with its history and the people who were instrumental in its earliest stages. Her executive priorities flowed from her personal philosophy of hospice, a philosophy embraced by her staff, who share her dedication to improving care of the terminal patient. Also in this segment are aspects of funding, decision making, and individual actor's participation in the planning process.

Q. I would like to talk with you about the broad area of PLANNING. We would like to look at some of the questions concerning the history of The Washington Hospice. When and with whom did the idea originate?

A. Well, it originated...its prehistory was actually a committee of the Episcopal Diocese in Washington. Members of the community who were affiliated with the Episcopal Church in Washington got together and began discussing the needs of the people of Washington concerning the idea of a hospice in the city. They spent a year looking at what was available and what wasn't. After a year they disbanded themselves, saying that there was a need for hospice, but the roots should be both interdenominational and interdisciplinary. So in the spring of 1977 a much more expanded group assembled, representing all sorts of disciplines and incorporated as "The Washington Hospice Society." That's the stage where I became involved.

Q. Who were some of the other people involved at that time?

A. There were nurses, doctors, lawyers...lots of people, and some lay people...taking in a number of professions. The whole array were people who simply had a gut feeling about the need for a hospice.

Q. What is the philosophy of The Washington Hospice Society? And what is your philosophy?

A. My philosophy is really a hospice philosophy. It involves caring for patients and their families using an interdisciplinary approach—with the help of doctors, nurses, social workers, clergy, trained volunteers, and many more people, professionals and nonprofessionals, who are brought in as the case warrants. The family is the unit of care. We're not simply treating a patient's disease but a whole person's sphere...his family or his extended family as the case may be. In particular, in our organization, we determined that home care would be our priority; for logistical reasons it is certainly easier to plan and easier to operate...and partly to see what the need would be for a facility given the existence of home care. That's not exactly a philosophy, but it is a policy, and the two seem to overlap. The other important thing about Washington Hospice concerns the city we're in...the plan of our organization is that Washington, D.C., is a heterogeneous unit, and we have special concerns and obligations to meet the needs of all kinds of people who live here. Although I must say that the organization was started by a group that was predominantly white and at least middle class, we have to reach out to a city that is mostly black with a number of other national and ethnic groups heavily represented. We do this in order to be as "multicultural" as possible. And that too becomes a philosophical consideration in the planning of the work that we are doing.

Q. When you first took office here, what did you see as some of your priorities?

A. Reaching out to the whole community was a priority.

Q. The total community?

A. Yes, and to make sure that we really were and remained a "grass-roots" organization and didn't get caught up in a great deal of health bureaucracy.

Q. What do you see as your priorities at the present time?

A. Some of the same things. I don't know that that has been accomplished yet, by any means. In a more immediate and practical way, we have just begun to give care, and so we have a priority of "working the bugs out of that system." We've started with a few patients and must raise the funds to expand our program so that eventually we can meet the total needs of the city. There is very little money or funding available for reimbursement of hospice services.

Q. Do you think that will change in the foreseeable future?

A. I think so. The reimbursement will change. I think that reimbursement in general is changing with all the interest in National Health Insurance. On a national level, I think there is some recognition of hospice. And, the government is about to grant contracts to various model hospices around the country, waiving Medicare and Medicaid restrictions so that they will get full reimbursement. As soon as enough data are generated, I do think that funding will begin to change. The problem is that hospice is so new that there have never been enough data upon which to base the cost effectiveness. The basic problem is unfamiliarity with hospice and the concept of hospice.

Q. In relation to the administrative function of PLANNING, how active would you say your organization is? How active would you say the following people are in the planning of the hospice: yourself, your staff, other professionals such as nurses, doctors, social workers? Does everyone have an "equal share of the pie" or, do some groups predominate in the planning function of this organization?

A. In some way, there is an equal kind of sharing. Obviously, some people predominate more as individuals than their disciplines simply because they have more time, or they're more available, or they've been doing it longer. There are people who are clearly more active. However, that doesn't divide along disciplines or anything else. It's really a matter of personality and circumstance. A hospice, unlike the more traditional health facility, has very different roots. It has roots in volunteerism and in a team approach. This also includes planning. People, at least at this stage, are working only out of conviction. It's not something from which one can become rich. With very few exceptions, it's not something from which one can acquire a great deal of prestige. It is a matter of your conviction concerning how people should be treated when they're dying. And those are the kind of people drawn to hospice. As a result, they take an active role. We have a board of directors and it is really a working board. People don't just sit back and let it happen. People have a very positive feeling about what we're doing and really take an active part in the planning and the setting of hospice policies and seeing that these policies are carried out.

Q. At the present time, should you have a final decision, who makes it? Do you make the final decisions?

A. The policy of this organization is set by the board and I certainly have an influence on them, but the bottom line does, indeed, rest with the board. In terms of operation or the day-to-day decisions of carrying out that policy, I make the final decision.

Organizing

Secondary to planning is the managerial function of organizing, which consists of determining the activities to be performed in an organization, grouping these activities, and assigning managerial authority and responsibility for them. In this domain the crucial questions that demand responses are: Who is to do what, and with how much authority? What is the environment like?

In determining the answers to these questions, such areas as organizational growth, structure, power, and authority must be explored. In addition, bureaucratic and community models and role determination necessitate analysis. Unlike most organizations, The Washington Hospice Society is characterized by an unusual structure. At present, this structure is elemental and departs markedly from the concept of bureaucracy. According to Lack and Buckingham 1978: 20, "the problem is to sustain hospice within the framework of American medical bureaucracy."

Care of the dying would seem to demand unique skills. Therefore, the task of staffing a hospice with persons who can effectively meet the needs of such "special" patients is formidable. The Washington Hospice emphasizes the importance and difficulty associated with the selection of its staff.

Q. In looking at organizational growth, the hospice movement seems to be literally "mushrooming" across the country. Do you think that this rapid proliferation is helpful, or do you believe it is a hindrance to the movement?

A. Well, it is sort of each. It is helpful in that suddenly all over the country people are talking about "hospice" and it is coming to the attention of the authorities in a way that it would not have if there had been only isolated hospices in certain areas of the country. In that respect, from a "consciousness-raising" point of view, it is helpful. On the other hand, it means that you have to be cautious because it is a very appealing idea, and one must be careful that people who are getting involved in hospices don't do it with a motive other than a humanistic one. Rapid growth has its pros and cons.

Q. How do your patients avail themselves to you? How do you get your referrals?

A. We accept a referral from anyone or from anywhere. We get referrals from doctors or other health professionals or practitioners; from discharge planners, hospitals, or any other kinds of services; from clergymen; from family or friends of the patient or the patient himself. Any phone call will do.

Q. You're open?

A. Entirely open.

Q. Could you tell me about the structure or the ORGANIZATION of The Washington Hospice Society—the organizational chart, the board, the governing body?

A. We have the simplest and flattest organizational chart you've ever seen. We have a board of directors of 27 working members, and they all serve on various committees to assist me with the various aspects of our development. I work for the board, and my staff consists of a couple of administrative assistants—one of whom is a volunteer. Then, there is my team of caregivers, including a part-time doctor, a nurse, a social worker, and a coordinator of volunteers. We also have trained volunteers and clergy who offer their services on a rotating basis. But we all work as a group. When we have case-planning meetings, everybody in the office participates. While the board doesn't participate on a day-to-day basis, very often members of the board who are experts in their fields are called on for planning or decision making or just discussing whatever the issue might be. We really operate in a very horizontal way, particularly because care is given by a team approach. There is no single authority, except that a doctor must sign for prescriptions, and he does that with the advice of the nurse. What we are seeing is true discipline interaction. I take part in helping plan for the care of patients, and my nurse takes part in helping me look for funds. It is a really "back and forth" kind of process.

Q. There are some places that tend to grow, particularly if they're popular, toward bureaucracy. Do you foresee this happening to The Washington Hospice Society?

A. I hope not. I hope I would have the good sense to get out if it did. Inevitably there will come a time when I don't know the day-to-day details of the patients. Presently, I can tell you as much about each of our patients as the nurse can. This is because we all take such an active role. As we grow, I suppose I'm going to have to lose track of those fine details. On the other hand, I look at other administrators in other health services and programs, and I realize that they spend a lot of time out of town. They also spend much of their time at meetings and giving talks. I have the feeling that this is because they're removed from the actual delivery of health care. Personally, I think such a situation would be unfortunate, and as far as I'm concerned, I don't intend to let that happen. I suppose there will be some diffusion with growth, but I hope that hospice doesn't become such a bureaucracy that the administrative side doesn't know what the delivery side is doing.

Q. In terms of staffing, I imagine that you will grow, and no doubt, growth is one of your goals. What do you see at the present time as some of your priorities in, and criteria for, the selection of your staff? I would guess that you would want very special people to work here.

A. That is correct. I think it takes a very special person to work in a hospice, and that is why I feel it is very hard to describe to anyone just what the credentials are for a hospice nurse. In fact, the government has requested a proposal for a training program for hospice nurses. We're also getting calls from people asking my opinion about what such credentials should be. I say "I can't tell you that" because I feel the most important factor is the gut feeling about the way people should be treated, about health care in this country, and about how people deserve to be cared for when they're dying. You can't teach someone this and you can't pick this up in training, but you can teach them to do virtually anything else. In looking for a hospice nurse or a hospice worker, I am, in fact, looking for people who are good solid practitioners, no matter what their discipline, and come highly recommended. But really, it depends on their gut feeling, their feeling about our community, and about the ramifications for a hospice in Washington, D.C.

Q. Part of what you're saying is that there are skills you can teach or at least try to teach someone, but compassion and caring cannot be taught.

A. That's right. You can sensitize people. I don't mean to say that someone is born either knowing or not knowing about caring or empathy, but you can pick this up in talking to people, learn from where they are coming, what is motivating them, and what kind of deep feelings they have about the kind of care hospice has to offer.

Q. Does everyone come through your office in terms of staff—your professional staff?

A. So far. Our staff is so small that everyone has, thus far. Maybe there will be a time when I won't be able to interview every last person. I must say, I would hate to think that that will happen.

Leading

Since the dawn of organizational life, the problem of leadership has perplexed managers and scholars alike. Despite the abundance of theories on the subject, "...no single theory has proven to be sufficiently inclusive to encompass all of the complexities involved in effective leadership" (Stoner 1978: 92). Yet leading remains a necessary component of organizational life and productivity. The critical question is: How does one get the employee to willingly meet the goals of the organization?

In a classic treatise on leadership, Tannenbaum and Schmidt have suggested two pertinent implications for the successful leader:

The first is that the leader is one who is keenly aware of those forces which are most relevant to his behavior at any given time. He accurately understands himself, the individual, the group he is dealing with and the environment in which he operates. Secondly, the successful leader is one who is able to behave appropriately in the light of these perceptions (1973: 180).

Leadership within The Washington Hospice begins with the executive director. Although most activity originates from a multidisciplinary team approach, major decisions are made with her knowledge and support. Internally motivated, this leader joins her staff in educating the public about the hospice concept. The established health care bureaucracy mandates that as a leader she must initiate necessary changes and use effective problem-solving strategy. A leader must also provide support for staff, and The Washington Hospice makes this provision. Equally important is lateral leadership support. To fulfill this need, this directory encourages a peer group exchange among other hospice managers.

Q. Concerning LEADERSHIP, how do you feel about your role? Would it be different, let's say, if you were a director at Georgetown University Hospital here in Washington? In other words, do you see your role as just another facet of health care, a managerial task, or do you think it's something very special because of hospice?

A. I don't know if I would function any differently if I were at Georgetown. I think partly that depends on a person's personality and how he conducts his affairs. But on the other hand, if I were at Georgetown, I would be dealing with a kind of "superstructure" that would be different from what I am dealing with here. This is the primary reason I'm not affiliated with an inpatient setting. I prefer our kind of setting; there's a great deal more intimacy in dealing with a whole staff or a whole program. In some respects, this is very special. Everybody here shares a special commitment to what we are doing. I'm not so sure the same would be true in a big institution. The people are there because they have simply found a job. They may be good at what they're doing and they may not be, but they do not show that "special" commitment. In terms of a hospice, our organization, such a commitment makes it very special. There's a certain relationship among us, the people working here.

Q. What do you feel motivates you?

A. A feeling about how people ought to be treated and the fact that people who are dying face the most traumatic time of their lives. What they deserve is *not* to have to give thought to any of the minutiae that absolutely plague people who are sick or who are not sick, who are just going through life. Things like dealing with financial issues and fighting for their sense of dignity and sense of control within the health care establishment. People shouldn't have to worry about these things when they're faced with their own death and, furthermore, I don't think they should have to suffer the kind of disorientation that everybody fears is going to happen in a hospital. I think that the health care providers, out of necessity, have become callous in their feelings concerning "what the man on the street feels" and *is* feeling when he goes into the hospital. When *I* go into a hospital, I get a little bit weak, and I'm in this business! I know that I, personally, would need a great deal of help if I were in a similar situation. I think that people who are in the much more traumatic situation of dying need and deserve tremendous support. They shouldn't be concerned with all the peripheral issues. I do not think that is the way they are treated in the more traditional health care delivery system. There ought to be an alternative.

Q. To the best of your knowledge, what do you feel motivates your staff?

A. The same feelings about how people should be treated.

Q. Where do your problems, either real or perceived, originate?

A. The problems don't come from my staff and, by and large, they don't come from the community, when we're speaking of individuals. They come from the established bureaucracy that has become so "entrenched" that so far, there is very little opening for the concept of hospice. When we had to get a "certificate of need" dealing with the whole planning process, we encountered incredible problems for reasons that I would never have guessed. First, there was the problem of educating people about hospice, but that is to be expected and that was all right. But what we really were was an "ally" of the consumer, and consumers dominated the committee! We were a consumer ally because we're a "grass-roots" organization, and I would have expected that they would have treated me warmly. I would have expected to be welcomed with open arms. We were not the establishment and we were not a big hospital with a big budget. But what happened was just the opposite. Those people were used to dealing with big hospitals, with their large expenditures, who were coming in asking to spend millions of dollars. Therefore, they were suspicious of us because we had such a small budget and because we talked about using volunteers. They insisted that we put in line items on our budget for volunteers. We just couldn't convince them that people were doing things out of the goodness of their hearts, and so it was a whole reversal of what you would have expected. We got the "certificate of need," and I'm sure we'll get by every other obstacle similar to that, but there is such an entrenchment of big spending in medicine that the people who should have been looking for the opposite couldn't see what was right in front of them. That is just one example, but the underlying fact is that hospice is *not* yet familiar to the establishment.

Q. Am I hearing you correctly then, that your problems arise from society?

A. Well, society in general is very responsive to hospice. In fact, the "grass-roots" segment of the population is behind our movement. But there is another aspect of society, i.e., the bureaucracy, and that is our source of trouble.

Q. Would it be fair to label what you have just described as the "health-care" bureacracy?

A. I suppose so.

Q. You have told us that the time is right for hospice and the "grass-roots" are ready. You seem to be right on the cutting edge of change theory with this movement. How, then, can change be initiated?

A. Partly through educational processes. And just by *being* and *doing*. The more publicity that hospice gets, the more likely we are to see change. You have probably seen numerous articles in newspapers around the country where people have shared personal accounts of deaths of their loved ones. People are out there just waiting for the alternative and, as it develops, are right behind it. In my opinion, what is really important to the hospice movement is to be sure that the consumer—the person who writes a letter and relates his own story—is always kept inside the movement. It must always remain a consumer-developed concept. With that kind of ideal, there will be change.

Q. With respect to your change efforts, do you foresee in the near future a full-time person whose job it is to provide this necessary societal education?

A. I hope so. Except that, in this organization thus far, we have allocated the majority of our expenditures for health care delivery. That is, the team members and the caregivers, rather than the administrative things, have been the recipient of funds. Eventually, I hope that we will come to a point where we will have a little bit of leeway, allowing room for community education and outreach as a full-time occupation. Right now, it is done partly through our volunteer component, a speaker's bureau, and through newsletters. And, of course, the board members do a large amount of it too, because they represent us in many areas. It doesn't receive, however, as much attention as it probably deserves.

Q. As a leader, to what extent are peer relationships important or helpful to you? Is there any peer group that you find particularly helpful?

A. I would say that is is helpful to talk with other hospice planners, and occasionally I get a chance to do that from meetings that I attend. Frequently, I just work on the phone in Washington because there are a number of other planners in the area. It is also very helpful to talk to other people who are involved in leadership positions in established home health care programs. For example, when I need to know the traditional way of doing things to comply with the government, it is helpful to be able to talk with someone who has been running a home health care agency for 20 years. I utilize those professionals who have more expertise than I have in certain specific areas.

Evaluating

Ideally, evaluation is an ongoing function that begins at the first identification of a need, continues throughout the planning and organizing phases, provides feedback to leadership, and projects into the future. "It results from systematic planning, involves a regular and comprehensive review of all phases of the program including the subsequent activities of those who participate, and serves as a mechanism for improving present and future programs and participants" (Staropoli and Waltz 1978: 83). The critical questions during this phase of management are: Did we reach our goal? Did *all* of us reach our goal? If not, what remediation is necessary to reach our goal?

The process of evaluation takes place on various levels within The Washington Hospice Society. Standards of care not only direct and appraise the team approach but also evaluate the quality of terminal care. The Washington program employs a system of identified dimensions where patients and their families are identified in relation to the caregiver's ongoing assessment.

Sound fiscal management is also an accurate indication of organizational success. Constraints and facilitators of the budget must also be subjected to analysis.

Q. Concerning the concept of EVALUATION, there are many hospice roles to be considered. There appears to be much overlapping of role function in work with the dying. You seem to suggest that this is indeed fact—not fiction or myth. Would you please comment further on this unique approach to patient care, true interdisciplinary care? How can this team approach be evaluated?

A. I consider it a goal to have things as interdisciplinary as possible. We try not to duplicate each other's efforts. We really attempt to complement each other in terms of evaluating our own patient care. We are doing an evaluation that will show how the various disciplines have had effects on areas of care that would not have traditionally been considered part of their specific function. For example, if my social worker goes into a home and finds a patient uncomfortable and suggests putting a sheepskin under him, and that gesture relieves some pain, then the social worker has had a physical effect on the patient. A clergyman in a similar situation might have done the same thing, which again affects the physiological aspects of that patient's care. We really consider this to be a priority—to see the disciplines interacting and looking for a "full picture" of the case. In evaluating this interaction, we hope to be able to track down and document the outcome of interdisciplinary service.

Q. Let us look at standards of care utilized by The Washington Hospice Society. What guides professional practice in this agency?

A. We are guided first of all by standards of good medical practice. More specifically, we are guided by the government's regulations and their requirements for certification as a home health agency. We must always comply with those kinds of things if there is any hope of getting reimbursement. We must write into our procedures all of those requirements. However, we have found that our own standards surpass most of the government regulations. We have concentrated our thought on the special kinds of care that our terminal patients require and have incorporated this thinking into our standards.

Q. How is the quality of care evaluated?

A. Any evaluation is subjective, but we do have a system where we track each patient and family according to half a dozen dimensions ranging from physical pain, emotional pain, some of the psychosocial aspects, spiritual aspects, and so forth. In this delineation, we have described levels where we can pinpoint the patient and the family. Each caregiver who makes a visit assesses the patient and the family with respect to these dimensions. From week to week we discuss the status of the patient and arrive at a consensus regarding future plans. Eventually we will be able to look and to see how a patient may have moved from one level to the next, and we draw some conclusions about the effect of our care on the progress being made. Because we are just beginning care and just beginning an evaluation process, we do not know what the pattern may be. We may be surprised, but at least we will be able to see the care we now deliver and compare it to what existed prior to hospice intervention.

Q. As the administrator, the executive director, would you share with us a bit about accountability in this organization? For example, for what do you hold the staff accountable?

A. The staff is accountable to the patients, to me, and to our organization for giving good care—for complying with all of the standards that constitute good care. There are some standards that are rather cut and dried. For example, we must have a physician sign a plan of care and he must review the case every 60 days. We are certainly held accountable for complying with various drug regulations. The staff is also responsible for upholding the spirit of this organization, and in that sense, they are accountable to the patients, the patients' families, and the larger community with which they come in contact.

Q. I guess if you are talking about the spirit of the hospice, they would also be accountable to themselves.

A. Yes. They all feel that rather deeply.

Q. For what, if anything, do you hold the patients, and/or the family accountable?

A. It varies from case to case regarding the capabilities of each patient and each family. In some cases we will hold them accountable for delivering a large part of the care and for reporting it. In other cases where this ideal is not possible, they are accountable only for knowing when and how to get in touch with us. In some cases, all we can count on is that we can write the telephone number and stick it on the wall somewhere so that the family member knows how to call our nurse in the middle of the night when they need her.

In one case, we were able to teach a sister how to suction a patient, change the colostomy bag, give injections of morphine every four hours, and do a great deal of the care while keeping track of it. So it is a matter of judging what the patient and family members are capable of doing. Often the patient, himself, can be responsible for much of his own care. In another case, we have a woman who is really ambulatory, but she needs someone with her all the time. Most of our activity has been to provide volunteer service on a regular basis. In this situation, we are holding her accountable for keeping track of when she is expecting help, which volunteer is coming next, if they did come, and so forth. It is not that we need to know the answers to these questions, but it is clear that she needs a particular task to do so that she will feel important and worthwhile in the whole process. It depends very much on the patient.

Q. From where does your funding come for The Washington Hospice Society?

A. Thus far, our funding has come almost exclusively from local sources. These include District of Columbia division of the Cancer Society, a number of local foundations, churches, and lots and lots of individuals.

Q. Obviously, this is a nonprofit organization. Do you expect it to remain one?

A. Yes. It will always be a nonprofit organization.

Summary

Although the hospice movement is relatively new in the United States, a wealth of material concerning the subjective component of caring for those who are entering the final stage of life exists already. Because the hospice concept has become a reality, the purpose of this interview with the executive director of The Washington Hospice Society was to pioneer a *new* perspective—managerial function. By employing the universal paradigm POLE, the early development of this particular program has been outlined within four segments or stages: planning, organizing, leading, and evaluating.

Of what importance are these distinctions? Their value is intrinsic to the success of any organization: goal setting and the explicit delineation and proper execution of activities taken to reach those goals. After a need is recognized, the planning begins. Organizing defines structure and helps to set priorities. Leadership mobilizes resources, and evaluation allows time to reflect, assess, and begin planning once again. POLE is a cycle: undirectional, uninterrupted, and dynamic.

The administrative elements of planning, organizing, leading, and evaluating provide a descriptive account of hospice development, whose effectiveness in communicating the hospice concept is as indisputable as the need for compassionate supporters. By bridging this gap between clinical concepts and managerial function, the hospice movement receives clearer focus.

References and Bibliography

Kazmier, L. J. 1974. *Principles of Management: A Programmed Instructional Approach,* *3rd ed.* New York: McGraw-Hill Book Company.

Lack, S. A. and R. W. Buckingham. 1978. *First American Hospice: Three Years of Home Care.* New Haven, Connecticut: Hospice, Inc.

Rubin, I. M., R. E. Fry, and M. S. Plovnick. 1978. *Managing Human Resources in Health Care Organizations: An Applied Approach.* Reston, Virginia: Reston Publishing Company.

Staropoli, C. J. and C. F. Waltz. 1978. *Developing and Evaluating Educational Programs for Health Care Providers*. Philadelphia: F. A. Davis.

Steiner, G. A. 1969. *Top Management Planning*. New York: Macmillan Company.

Stoner, J. A. F. 1978. *Management*. Englewood Cliffs, New Jersey: Prentice-Hall.

Tannenbaum, R. and W. H. Schmidt. 1973. "How to Choose a Leadership Pattern." *Harvard Business Review* (May-June) 51:162-80.

Acknowledgment

The interview cited above was conducted with Ms. Susan Silver, Executive Director (1979) of the Washington Hospice Society. The authors wish to express appreciation for her cooperation.

Part II

Ethical and Human Issues in Terminal Care

6

A Right to Die?

Richard A. Metz

I

The practice of medicine is undergoing continual change as new treatments are devised for known and new entities. Treatment that today is considered extraordinary, will be ordinary tomorrow; one need only consider the field of organ transplantation. While the medical profession is aware of these varied advances, and the general population has come to expect more and better care, a problem of significant proportions is created. It has become more difficult to cease treatment because of an ever-rising community standard of care. And because the law has not been able to keep pace with the changing milieu of the practice of medicine, the physician often finds himself in, or feels himself to be in, a paradoxical situation.[1]

    Can he cease treatment on the patient who is terminally ill, is on the respirator, and is dependent upon the respirator, without being accused of murder? Can the physician agree to a patient's request to cease treatment, or the family's if the patient is unable to speak for himself, without being accused of murder? The physician is forced to face these questions more and more frequently. Yet he has no firm guidelines to follow from his own professional ethics, the law, theology, or general societal morality and ethics.

This paper is predicated on the following: that there is a right to die; that this is an area of societal concern that is currently being confronted. Since the extant case and statutory law is minimal on the direct question, the courts will be the sources of guidance until statutes are passed, but to do this, the courts will have to attempt an interpretation of society's feelings and rely on societal agents to guide their decisions.

While I shall make every effort to be impartial in this presentation, it is only fair to acknowledge that I am biased toward the affirmative in regard to allowing cessation of treatment.

To discuss a right to die, one must define death, life, and living in more detail than the unabridged dictionary provides. Living is "engaging in mentation."[2] It is a dynamic state in both the biological and sociological sense. It is more than mere existence and the functioning of a natural entity. Man is a social being, thriving on interactions with other human beings and also with other forms of living things—plants and animals.

Life can be considered to be the biological counterpart to living. Life exists as long as the tissues, organs, and the component cells function to carry on respiration, metabolism, and excretion.[3] Life is purely a physical series of events; it is not interactive except to what is internal to the organism. Living is absolutely dependent upon life, but life can exist without living. It is this issue that will become important in evaluating the question of a right to die.

II

The issue at hand truly becomes the attempt to provide a definition of death that can be objectively applied in all cases and never found to be in fault. It is a medical question that requires the setting of standards, the application thereof, and the interpretation of the application. This is the role of the physician, who may (have to), and has, turned to the law for legal support.

No state has developed a definition of death nor have they established criteria for when it occurs. It is a retrospective fact: the patient *has* died. The same medical advances that can save a life and allow living to continue make it more difficult for the physician to say that death has occurred or that death *is* occurring.

From varying sources it can be learned that death is the cessation of life; the process of dying; the point of time when processes become irreversible or when the soul leaves the body for final judgment; or, "human life continues for as long as its vital functions, as distinguished from the simple life of organs, manifest themselves without the help of artificial processes."[4]

On the basis of the lack of statutory definitions of death, it is often stated that you are dead when a physician says you are dead. While this is imprecise, not truly satisfying, and considered to be overly physical, it may be the best definition from the standpoint of modern medicine. Remember, what causes death today may be reversible tomorrow. To strengthen the patient-physician-family relationships, it would also serve to do what is best in the minds of those most concerned and related to the patient.

Biologically, life is dependent upon the circulatory and respiratory systems' proper functioning, upon signals delivered through the sympathetic and autonomic nervous systems. This is the basis of the definition of death as contained in Black's Law Dictionary.[5] The vital signs of temperature, blood pressure, and respiration as the determinants of life were the only basis for early medicine. Modern equipment, when attached to a failing body, can maintain the vital signs almost forever. Yet, without such apparatus, the vital signs would cease.[6]

This becomes the crux of the dilemma facing the physician: does one provide for the continuation of the living of the person, or only of his life? Note that society says of a murderer that he has taken a life, without which there can be no living. And I am repulsed by the thought of a person who has been shot, who continues to be alive but is unable to continue "living." Yet in many states, there is no statutory mechanism by which the physician can discontinue the equipment maintaining life.[7]

Such an action requires a basis for the declaration of death that is unrelated to the respiratory and circulatory systems.

This has led to the need to define the occurrence of death in an alternate manner, the formulation of a definition of brain death, the prime source of which is the so-called "Harvard criteria."[8] The advancements in medicine and the medical equipment that society values so much and expects so much from are beginning to be questioned because of their financial impact. There is a need to recognize that respiratory and circulatory failure are not the only possible means to establish that death has occurred. Death should and can be recognized when the brain has suffered irreversible damage, just as it can and should be recognized when the heart or any other vital organ is irreversibly damaged. These criteria provide an objective basis for a physician to state that death has occurred. They are designed to allow their application with or without the use of special medical equipment; the local standards are to be applied by the physician in reaching his decision.[9] It is evident by the legal decisions found that the judicial acceptance of this new standard is slow in coming.[10] But as various state statutes are passed codifying "brain death," it will become more acceptable to society in general.

Besides providing a medical basis for understanding death, it is also necessary to discuss the meaning of life and death in the sociological terms by which members usually respond to the concept. That death is universal and inevitable goes without saying; yet it is also universal that death is a taboo topic. Most people cannot conceive, or are unwilling to conceive, their own nonexistence.[11] Rather than openly accept the concept of their own death, they make every attempt to deny that this will eventually occur. (Witness the people who refuse to prepare their own will.)

Death is often seen as failure by the medical profession. It means to the layman that an existing set of relationships has ended. The problem of accepting the finality of the event is alleviated by the rituals that are followed when there is death. Is the funeral for the dead or the living?

These attitudes create impediments to the acceptance that at some point in time death has or will occur and that it should be accepted and welcomed: "A dying man needs to die, as a sleepy man needs to sleep, and there comes a time when it is wrong, as well as useless, to resist."[12]

Until such an attitude reaches *expressed* general acceptance, the question of a right to die may never be fully discussed and responded to.

Man has ascribed many roles to the heart—the repository of the soul, and so forth.[13] The linkage between this and the use of respiratory and circulatory failure as providing the means of establishing clinical death is obvious. But as medicine has grown and the secular nature of society takes increasing precedence over the nonsecular aspects, we find that this special role, which is greatly philosophical and theological, gives way to more factual, possibly utilitarian criteria for determining that death has occurred.[14] Because man is different from animal life forms, because of the development of the brain, it is extremely logical to use its status in the determination of death. This is no different from the references to the heart during the early days.

III

Suicide and euthanasia, related as they are to the topic, are special topics in their own right. They are briefly discussed for purposes of clarity and completeness.

Statutory response to suicide is varied in this country but is primarily based on the English Common Law, which makes it or its attempt a crime.[15] Suicide is an overt act and always appears to be the result of a conscious decision.[16] Whether the act is rational may or may not be determinable owing to the subjective nature of the term *rational*. This raises the privacy issue, both medically and legally. We all have a constitutional right to be left alone, unless we are proved, or are believed, to be a threat to another or to ourself. (The former is not for discussion here.) Society has determined and codified that a decision to take one's own life is sufficient proof of being a self-threat.

The mental processes by which a person arrives at the decision of suicide may very well be based on events that, when viewed at a later perspective, may be manageable. When this is the case, interventions to provide such opportunities are valid and valuable. Yet what about the case where such interventions do not provide a new or different perspective, or do confirm the decision of suicide, should there not be a right to enforce this decision in private?[17]

A collateral issue, and one that can and should override the right of privacy, is the existence of person(s) dependent upon the contemplator. If such dependents were acquired voluntarily and the act of suicide places their burden on others or the state, a reasonable case can be made that this is not an act affecting only one person. Now there is a larger interest. However, should a person be forced to continue a "miserable existence?"

Obviously, the discussion can proceed pro and con on many levels, regardless of the laws in effect. How does one prosecute the perpetrator of a successful suicide? Furthermore, if it is unsuccessful, the criminal is the victim. Has society truly been injured?

A somewhat different issue is raised when a person is asked to assist another in committing suicide. Has such a person committed a crime and is he liable for prosecution under the homicide or manslaughter statutes? This raises the question of assuring that those who choose to live do not fall prey to a murderer, who would then claim immunity by a defense of suicide. There are cases related to such actions for review.[18]

Euthanasia[19] means literally "a good death" and usually entails the involvement of others. It can be, for the patient in a hospital, the result of an omission of care or of the commission of an act that becomes the event prior to death. It is not, or may not, be the proximate cause of death. As stated in several books consulted during my research, it is an acknowledged fact by those who work in a medical setting. It is an act that is "committed" today, and one that should remain private to the family-doctor-patient relationship.

Euthanasia should also be separated from the mercy-killing concept. The former implies an understanding between the patient and doctor about a point in time when the patient no longer consents to medical treatment. Mercy killing implies a decision by some member of the medical team that is rendering care, without an express statement (current or past) from the patient or the family. Certain rights of patients exist that lend support to a right of euthanasia: (1) the right to be informed when ill so that valid decisions can be made; (2) the right to refuse treatment as long as it is not harmful to others; (3) the right to refuse treatment and know the refusal will be honored even if one becomes incompetent.[20]

The difference between suicide and euthanasia may be a semantic one when considered in this light and when the patient is competent to consent. But what about the patient unable to give consent who has expressed his desires in the past? Should the physician not be able to rely on this information just as he can accept their consent as valid for treatment?

Euthanasia always involves others and hence can lead to the legal difficulties of aiding, or not preventing or assisting, the commission of a crime. The few court cases available to date indicate that the juries are swayed by motivation.[21] Euthanasia is usually applied to the person who has entered the acute phase of an illness and, more often than not, is not able to express his desires. Those who proceed to "implement" euthanasia are doing so based either on past desire or their own wishes or beliefs of what the person wanted.

Suicide is usually thought of as an act by one who is not in an acute medical crisis. Although the psychological aspects of suicide should never be discounted and can often be dealt with to eliminate the felt need to complete the act, it may, as previously stated, be an objective and valid desire.

This division may be criticized as being artificial. To provide an example, the magazine section, *New York Times*, March 18, 1979, is cited. The author, at age 67, was faced with a diagnosis of cancer of the colon and the decision of whether or not to have surgery. Not only did he deal with the disease itself and the decision regarding surgery (eventually performed), but he also planned for his own suicide to avoid the following situation:

Closely monitored by family and caretakers they (already physically or mentally incapacitated) lack any access to any effective means of suicide.

He cited cases that supported this statement and expounded on the role of the cancer patient vis-à-vis the physician:

The surgical option is too often presented to the patient as if it were not an option but a forgone conclusion...Thus, at the very beginning of their careers as patients...(they) are deprived of an invaluable privilege of the human condition: the opportunity to plot their own course.

What he is asking for is an alternate to the usual cancer options of surgery or painful death. Such an option is the right to refuse surgery "and then to terminate it (life) in your own way at a moment of your own choosing."

When he discussed his plans, he received support, not only from his sons (his wife had died several years earlier of cancer), but also from friends and medical professionals. Not only was the support moral, but also it existed to the extent of wanting to give the injection and to be present at the appointed time. The problem of the potential prosecution of those present was felt to be minimal owing not only to the changing attitudes of prosecutors but also to the "sympathy and human concerns of jurors." This situation may be idealistic, and obviously those involved were willing to take such a risk, but I suspect that a decision similiar to that rendered in the Repouille case would be given. (This case could be an example of a mercy killing except that the patient is making the decision and appears absolutely rational, and his decision is in lieu of accepting medical care. The fact that another might actually give the fatal injection should not change the name of the act by which death occurred.)

IV

Virtually all of the people who will be requesting the cessation of extraordinary life support systems, or on whose behalf such a request will be made, will be patients in a hospital. If not, they may be in a nursing home or be a cancer patient who has elected to die at home. A common thread among all is that at some point a consent for treatment had to have been given. The following is a brief discussion of the law regarding the consent for medical treatment.[22]

Before a doctor or member of a hospital's staff can render treatment to a patient (except when a clearly defined emergency exists), a specific, informed consent must be given by the patient or the authorized guardian. To proceed without consent represents a technical battery on the part of both the hospital and the physician. These consents can be both written or oral, expressed or implied, but obviously the former in each set is the preferred. The implied consent is going to be held valid only where the patient voluntarily submitted to the procedure and the nature of the risks was readily apparent. In all other situations, an expressed, written consent is necessary to show that the patient or guardian was properly informed:

That consent obtained after the patient has been given sufficient information so that he understands *substantially* the value of the procedure to be performed, the *risks* and *consequences* thereof, and the courses of actions open to consideration other than the contemplated procedure.

The doctor is required to give the information that will allow the formulation of an intelligent decision, and not necessarily the decision that the doctor wants. The hospital has a concurrent responsibility in that setting to ensure that a proper consent has been obtained by the person(s) responsible.

Where a minor is involved, the courts have generally upheld the right of the parents to withhold treatment, especially if there is no emergency present. For the doctor or hospital to proceed would create liability for a battery. The basis is that English Common Law did not recognize the denial of medical care as the equivalent of child neglect. It was based on the natural right of custody.

Given the differences in the nature of society then and today, as evidenced by many factors, including child labor laws, a change in the law would be expected. There are state laws that modify the natural right of custody, but they are based on one or more of the following: the existence of an immediate danger, the risk to health, the effect upon the social and psychological development of the child, the balancing of the risks and benefits of the procedure and, where sufficient maturity is present, the personal wishes of the child.

When an incompetent adult is at issue, if there has been an adjudication of such, there is a guardian extant and consent is not an issue. If there is doubt as to competency, and this and the following must be a decision by the physician, a decision is made on whether the patient has the ability to understand and appreciate the nature of the procedure and the consequences thereof.

It is well accepted that a competent adult can refuse medical treatment regardless of the basis for refusal. Whereas cases are cited later on that generally show that a court will grant a petition ordering treatment on an adult, where a minor is involved, there are cases where this was not done (*e.g.*, 294 A2nd 372).

V

The premier case is that of Karen Ann Quinlan, in which the family petitioned to remove the respirator from their daughter. Unfortunately, the information that was presented to the general public did not reflect the facts of the case. I start here with a summary of the situation as it existed, and deal with the issues raised in the appellate courts.[23]

Karen Ann Quinlan was 20 years old at the time the medical drama began. While with friends at a party she apparently ingested an unknown combination of drugs and alcohol leading to the eventual and current comatose state. There is no evidence of malpractice.

Treatment was instituted to no avail, as were attempts to wean her from the respirator. After some period of time, the patient's parents petitioned the court to be appointed as her guardian. Both the hospital and the physicians involved were reluctant, or unwilling, to comply with their request to remove the respirator, although there was no disagreement about her status and chances of recovery.

The Equity Court trial, heard by Judge Muir, appointed Mr. Quinlan guardian of her property but appointed another as guardian of her person. Judge Muir's ruling was that the respirator could not be removed. This was then appealed. The following issues were discussed by the Supreme Court of New Jersey (355 A^{2nd} 647) in reaching their decision: Mr. Quinlan should be appointed the guardian of the person of Karen Ann Quinlan as well as her property; that under the condition cited, the respirator could be removed; that no civil or criminal liability could be assessed against any of the participants to such an act.

The court found no judicial basis for Mr. Quinlan *not* to be appointed as guardian of person and property. There is always a judicial preference for the next of kin, even when the person involved is not a minor.

Throughout the trial, religious beliefs were intimately involved.

Karen Ann Quinlan was in a Catholic hospital, and the family was accepted as being religious by both the court and the New Jersey Catholic Conference, which submitted an amicus curiae brief. Yet this issue itself would not provide an answer. The court's summary:

The right to religious belief is absolute but conduct in pursuance thereof is not wholly immune from governmental restraint.[24]

An issue of cruel and unusual punishment was raised in the plaintiff's case and almost summarily dismissed as unapplicable in all but penal cases.

The right of privacy issue, as it relates to medical interventions, found great favor with the court, and a multitude of United States Supreme Court cases have recognized this right as being constitutional. Over the years this right has been extended to cover the right to decline medical treatment. (At this point the abortion issue could be raised. It was to the extent of the cases cited therein.)

Two important issues are now raised. The first is that as the degree of bodily invasion increases, as compared to the chances for recovery, there is a concurrent increase in the right of the patient to say, "*Stop.*" This right devolves to the guardian when the patient is no longer competent. The second issue is the state's claim to a right to do all to preserve life. The parents stated that Karen Ann Quinlan had previously expressed her wish never to be maintained in a vegetative state. "It should not be discarded solely on the basis that her condition prevents her exercise of the choice."[25]

The court spent much time dealing with the medical issues, as well as the legal aspects of the practice of medicine. Briefly, one should note an earlier distinction between the self-infliction of bodily harm, the discontinuance of artificial life-supporting equipment, and the effect upon the medical decision to institute life support.

The role and right of medical discretion becomes crucial. While this is accorded to medicine by society as codified in the state statutes, it is also based on the "moral judgments of the community at large." There is a large history of case law that accepts this and the role of the "prevailing standards," and the Supreme Court did not fault Judge Muir for his decision. It did, however, declare that an evaluation was appropriate.

The special role assigned to the physician includes the making of moral and ethical judgments that may not always have a legal basis. Yet the court did not feel that application to a court for concurrence in similar actions would be best. It would prove cumbersome and should remain within a patient-doctor-family relationship. A now prominent phase was then established:

The evidence convinces us that the focal point of decision should be the prognosis as to the reasonable possibility of return to cognitive and a sapient life, as distinguished from the forced continuance of that biological vegetative existence to which Karen seems to be doomed.[26]

Because of the threat of criminal liability, the court was forced to face this issue. Criminal liability was summarily dismissed as the cause of Karen Ann Quinlan's death, if it occurred after the respirator was removed. Death would be from natural causes and, therefore, not a homicide. Further, "even if it were regarded as homicide, it would not be unlawful." The latter is true because it was the result of the termination of treatment as a matter of the right of privacy.

The final decision was given as follows:

Upon the concurrence of the guardian and family of Karen, should the responsible attending physicians conclude that there is no reasonable possibility of Karen's ever emerging from her present comatose condition to a cognitive, sapient state and that the life-support apparatus now being administered to Karen should be discontinued, they shall consult with the hospital "Ethics Committee" or like body of the institution in which Karen is then hospitalized. If that consultative body agrees that there is no reasonable possibility of Karen's ever emerging from her present comatose condition to a cognitive, sapient state, the present life-support system may be withdrawn and said action shall be without any civil or criminal liability therefor on the part of any participant, whether guardian, physician, hospital or others. We herewith specifically so hold.[27]

The court also conjoined the seemingly unrelated issues of the medical malpractice crisis that existed at the time: euthanasia and homicide. It was acknowledged that the malpractice crisis may have led the attending physician and hospital to continue the respirator, not in the best interest of the patient but in effect in their own interest of avoiding litigation.[28] By not agreeing in private with the family as the traditional patient-doctor-family relationship would have dictated, the matter had drawn the potential for a homicide charge. Had the physician accepted the "death with dignity" concept, his actions would not have become constrained.

The uncertainty of the expressed law in such cases did not aid the situation. Once public, however, the physician and the family were left with no choice but to petition the court.

The final decision provided protection to the medical community in two ways: by stating a procedure that could be followed as stipulated by an ethics committee and by defining the relationship between the act desired and the potential for civil and criminal liability.

The court further introduced the role of "the common moral judgment" as a means of reaching a decision in such cases. This illustrated not only a proper role for the court but also the limitations of such a role, and the interrelationship of this role and the "common moral judgment."[29]

It is an expression of a nation's character, shaped by education, superstition, material needs, and the press of copying. It can be informed by ethical principles and by scientific facts but it cannot be controlled by them alone.[30]

VI

The case of *Repouille vs. U. S.* (165 F2nd 152) (1947)[31] is one of the request by the appellee to become a naturalized citizen. Prior to the filing of such a petition and thereafter, he was conceded to be a man of good moral character, a good father and provider. The incident that led to his being rejected was that he put to death a son of thirteen years. The reason was:

He suffered from birth from a brain injury which destined him to be an idiot and a physical monstrosity. . . . The child was blind, mute and deformed. He had to be fed; the movements of his bladder and bowels were involuntary. . . .

While the jury found him guilty of manslaughter in the second degree (he had been tried in the first degree) they did so with the recommendation of "utmost clemency." The judge, who apparently agreed, handed down a sentence of five to ten years but placed the defendant on probation, from which he was discharged.

The court had to rule on the meaning of the phrase "good moral character" (It did so, I believe, reluctantly.) The court found that the order for naturalization be denied. It was done, though, so that a second petition could be filed at a later date.

The case of *Griswold v State of Connecticut* (85 S. Ct. 1678) (1965) (one of many repeatedly found and cited) concerns the violation of a 1958 state statute prohibiting the giving of "information, instruction and medical advice to married persons as to the means of preventing contraception." The relevancy of the case to this topic is the issue of privacy as it is protected by the various amendments to the Constitution and (briefly mentioned) the professional relationship between a physician and his patient.[32]

The right of privacy, while not explicitly stated in the Constitution, is found to exist from several sources. The court's primary conceptualization comes from the "penumbra" of the First Amendment, "privacy is protected from governmental intrusion." They found further support for the right of privacy as it related to the question at hand in the Third Amendment, the Fourth Amendment ("right of the people to be secure in their persons, houses, papers, and effects, against unreasonable searches and seizures"), the Fifth Amendment, and the Ninth Amendment ("the enumeration in the Constitution, of others [rights] retained by the people").[33]

The Fourth and Fifth Amendments, as they have been described in *Boyd v. U. S.* (116 U. S. 616, 630; S. 6 Ct. 524, 532; 29 L. Ed. 746), are protectors "of the sanctity of a man's home and the privacies of life."[34]

Several references were made to the concept of "the traditions and conscience of our people." This concept provides a basis for the court to decide cases rather than rely on their own notions when the answer to the question at hand cannot be directly determined. While the role of the courts is not to "substitute their social and economic beliefs for the judgment of the legislative bodies...,"[35]

Furthermore, they described the limitation on the right of a state to regulate activities involving personal liberties as requiring the "showing (of) a subordinating interest which is compelling." The law must be "necessary...to the accomplishment of a permissible state policy."[36]

This statement was enhanced by Justice Harlan in a concurring decision by the following:

"Specific" provisions of the Constitution, no less than "due process," lend themselves as readily to "personal" interpretations by judges whose constitutional outlook simply keeps the Constitution in supposed "tune with the times."[37]

One of the expressed purposes of the Connecticut statute was to enhance other laws prohibiting illicit sexual relationships. Yet if this was the purpose, why was there not a ban on the importation of such devices into the state or on their possession? This paradox or contradiction was cited by Justice White.

The dissenting opinion, in discussing the physician-patient relationship, drew a distinction between the protections of free speech from the First and Fourth Amendments and the protection to be accorded such actions and physical activities.[38]

But are the two really separable? I would argue not, especially when a physician-patient relationship is present.

The right of the court to consider cases on the basis of the "(collective) conscience of our people" was belittled as not within the realm of the Constitution but has been "bestowed on the court by the court."[39] It is my belief that when a question has been presented to the court for a decision and accepted by the court, all relevant facts (statutory and otherwise) should be considered by the court in arriving at a decision. How else can we maintain a dynamic set of laws to guide a contemporary society by a past that is valuable and yet by new concepts that should not be overruled? Judicial decisions, because of the political realities of legislatures, may be the only way to keep the basic rules of society concurrent with social, economic, and technological advances.

A recent Florida case is related. Abe Perlmutter was suffering from Lou Gehrig's disease[40] and wanted to be removed from the respirator. The following is a summary of the facts and the appellate decision.[41]

Lou Gehrig's disease, once diagnosed, usually leads to death within two years. Regarding Mr. Perlmutter, it is important to remember his physical status: incapable of movement; required the respirator for breathing; required great effort to speak; legally competent.

Based on his medical status, it was expected that if and when the respirator was removed (which the patient had already attempted several times) he would live only for one hour. The family supported Mr. Perlmutter's decision, as did, apparently, the hospital and attending physicians. Yet because of the lack of statutory guidance and past case history, they did not feel free to concur with the discontinuance of the respirator.

The trial court's final decision, which supported Mr. Perlmutter, was:

In the exercise of his *right of privacy*, [he] may remain in defendant hospital or leave said hospital, free of the mechanical respirator now attached to his body and all defendants and their staffs are restrained from interfering with plaintiff's decision.

The Broward State Attorney appealed on the following grounds:

The state has an overriding duty to protect life; the termination of supportive care equals unlawful homicide or manslaughter

The plight of the patient, his family, the hospital, and its physicians are hereby further exemplified.

The appellate court affirmed the trial court's decision, using a 1977 Massachusetts case (to be discussed) and the Quinlan case for further support. Their decision can be summarized as follows:

1) Perlmutter has a constitutional right of privacy to refuse treatment.
2) The State's interest in preserving life is supportable if the disease was curable, but where such is not the case, this interest cannot be superior to that of the patient.
3) The abandonment issue, so often raised in blood transfusion cases, is not applicable, because all of his family are adults (Perlmutter was over 60 years of age).
4) This is not a case of suicide, because the cause of death is natural, not "unnatural," and is not self-induced.
5) No patient is required to accept "fruitless surgery." Furthermore, the state's general contention that the patient cannot refuse treatment is invalid since, in this case, the patient is competent.
6) The preservation of medical ethics, while a most valid concern, is not in jeopardy, since medicine must be concerned not only with the prolongation of life but also with the comforting of the dying.
7) If informed consent has any meaning, the petition is a valid one.

Number five above is based on the Quinlan decision.

For these reasons, the appellate court found for Mr. Perlmutter, required that any appeals be filed promptly, but did not certify the case to the State Supreme Court. A separate concurring decision faulted the latter stipulation because it would not further the issuance of a judicial statement on these acts, especially because the decision is limited to a case of similar specific fact and the competency of the patient.

The case of *Roe v Wade* (93S.Ct. 705 [1973])[42] has been frequently cited as further support based on the right of privacy. It arose from the claim of a pregnant woman that the Texas abortion statutes were unconstitutional. This decision resulted in a partial affirmation and reversal of the Texas law that prohibited any abortion at any stage except to save the life of the mother.

The decision allowed the following as being a proper exercise of state function in regard to this issue: (1) that prior to the end of the first trimester, the decision to end a pregnancy is a matter between the woman and her physician; (2) that subsequent to the first trimester, the state may establish regulations reasonably related to maternal health; (3) that subsequent to the viability of the fetus the state may regulate and proscribe.

This case is cited, not because of its being an abortion case, but because of the statements made regarding privacy and the role of the physician, as follows:

1) The right of personal privacy does exist under the Constitution. This law was expounded in much the same language as, and cited in, the Griswold case (85 S.Ct. 1678 (1965). They did go on to acknowledge the state's interest in safeguarding health and the maintenance of proper standards, but such interest could not override the right of privacy.

2) "Where certain fundamental rights are involved, regulations limiting these rights may be justified only by a compelling state interest and the legislative enactments must be normally drawn to express only legitimate state interests."

3) The right of the physician to administer medical care according to his professional judgments cannot be abridged unless there is an important state interest involved.

Hence, the basis for the standards cited above can be understood. (I also believe that the basis is reflected in the other cited cases.)

The case of *Superintendent of Belchertown State School v Joseph Saikewicz* (370 NE[2nd] 417 (1977) was amply quoted in the Perlmutter case.[43] Saikewicz, 67 years of age, had been a resident of the school since 1923. He had developed leukemia and the issue was obtaining consent for chemotherapy. A petition for the appointment of a guardian ad litem was granted, the guardian subsequently determining that no treatment would be best, as follows: the disease was incurable; the patient was unable to cooperate with the treatment; the patient would not understand the side effects of chemotherapy, especially the pain; and certain death would be less painful without treatment.

The state raised four issues under which the authorization for treatment should be granted. Only two were accepted as potentially applicable: the protection of the interests of innocent third parties and the prevention of suicide.

Regarding the preservation of life, the state had a legitimate interest where a cure is possible. A distinction was made between care that prolongs life versus that which is life saving. The fourth issue was the maintenance of the integrity of medical ethics, which was found inapplicable because of a patient's right to refuse treatment at any time, especially when there are no dependents involved.

Because Saikewicz was an incompetent, two issues were raised: must medical treatment always be given and, if there is a choice, how is it to be made? The court responded that there is a choice due to the basic dignity of human life and that the incompetent have the same rights as the competent. The Quinlan decision was of considerable support to this court although the issue was not equivalent. The goal, "to determine with as much accuracy as possible the wants and needs of the individual involved," was available to the Quinlan court based on the testimony of the parents. In this case, Saikewicz was never able to communicate.

The final decision established the following: (1) a person has the right to refuse treatment in terminal cases; (2) this right extends to the mentally incompetent; (3) the substituted judgment doctrine is valid and applicable; and (4) the law recognizes the individual interest in preserving the inviolability of the person.

The court wanted to establish a framework for deciding such cases in the future. Unlike *Quinlan*, where the court felt that such decisions should not always be presented to them, they wanted all like decisions to be made or reviewed by the court. Such feelings may be based on the desire to ensure that the judgments are in accordance with the feelings of the population, based on the following idea:

The law always lags behind the most advanced thinkers. It must wait until the theologians and moral bodies and events have created some common ground, some consensus.[44]

There are many cases reported concerning the administration of blood for transfusions to Jehovah's Witnesses. While the issue of the right to consent for treatment is fairly well understood, these cases would appear to provide the basic guidance to courts on the topic at hand. The following are summaries of the pertinent cases found:[45]

In Erickson v Dilgard (252 NYS[2nd] 705 [1962]), the New York State Supreme Court held that an adult patient can refuse blood transfusions, regardless of the extant medical opinion, even if it means the taking of one's own life. Especially when the patient is competent, such a decision is a matter of judgment, and the penal laws are not applicable.

In Re: Ricky Ricardo Green (292 A[2nd] 387 [1971]) the court ruled that between a parent and child the state has no interest that overrules the religious beliefs of the family regarding medical treatment, if the child's life is not immediately impaired. Furthermore, at a certain age prior to majority (in this case age 16), the wishes of the child should be ascertained.

In *Raleigh-Fitkin-Paul Morgan (etc.) Hospital v Anderson* (201 A[2nd] 537 [1964]) the court felt justified in ordering the woman to have the transfusions because her life and that of her child's were too intertwined to provide a separate ruling on each.

In *Applic. of the Pres. and Directors of Georgetown College, Inc.* (331 F[2nd] 1000 [1963]) the court did order transfusions refused on religious grounds by patient and spouse. There was a seven month old child in the family. They also ruled that the courts can order compulsory medical treatment for children of a serious illness and for adults if there is a contagious disease present. In the case of the latter, the usual religious exemption does not apply.

In Re: Brooks Estate (205 NE[2nd] 435 [1965]), the court voided the appointment of a conservator in a case where the patient and spouse had specifically released the hospital and physician from liability owing to their refusal to have a transfusion. It was found to have violated their constitutional rights regarding religion and beliefs. There were no minor children involved, and there existed no danger to society.

Other cases were found that supported the following: privacy,[46] acknowledgment of a minor's constitutional rights,[47] the issue of right and privileges vis-à-vis constitutional rights,[48] (specifically on the abortion issue, which cases have provided the basis for a portion of this discussion) the right to an abortion also applies to the minor.[49]

In 1976, California enacted a new section to their Health and Safety Code entitled the Natural Death Act.[50] Although similar legislation has been introduced elsewhere in the country, including Florida (by Representative Sackett, a physician), none has been passed. It can reasonably be assumed, therefore, that this law will be the model for those that may be proposed elsewhere.

A discussion of the statute by section is appropriate, not only since it is the first in the country, but also because these sections highlight points raised elsewhere.

Not only do adults have the right to consent to medical care, but such rights include the withdrawal of such consent. This section, and the others to follow, are based on the existence of a *terminal* condition in an adult only. This right is further enhanced, or has become of greater significance, because of the prolongation of life that is possible by modern medicine, with concomitant loss of dignity and increase in suffering.

A definition[51] of a life-sustaining procedure is given that, when applied retrospectively and prospectively to Karen Ann Quinlan, is reflective of one of the limits to the law:

Utilizes mechanical or other artificial means to sustain, restore, or supplant a vital function, which when applied to a qualified patient, would serve only to artificially prolong the moment of death and where in the judgment of the attending physician death is imminent whether or not such procedures are utilized. Life sustaining procedure shall not include the administration of medication or other performance of any medical procedure deemed necessary to alleviate pain.

The limitation referred to is the last sentence. Karen Ann Quinlan is being given medication to prevent infection. Apparently such medication would not have been considered within the purview of this law and could not be discontinued without liability. Even in such cases, this aspect of medical care is considered ordinary.

California's Natural Death Act's definition of terminal condition should also be noted:

"Terminal condition" means an incurable condition caused by injury, disease, or illness which, regardless of the application of life-sustaining procedures, would, within reasonable medical judgment, produce death, and where the application of life-sustaining procedures serve only to postpone the moment of death of the patient.

The authorized directive to a physician provides in essence:[52]

1. Being competent, the signor makes known his/her desire not to have his/her life artificially prolonged.
2. Terminal status is to be confirmed by two physicians to the effect that death would occur regardless of medical intervention.
3. The directive is an "expression of legal right to refuse treatment."[53]
4. If the patient is pregnant, the directive is void during such pregnancy.[54]

As the patient's right to refuse medical treatment is acknowledged throughout the statute, evidenced by the revoking of consent, so may a properly signed directive be withdrawn "without regard to his mental state or competency,"[55] by a destruction of the directive, its written revocation, or a verbal statement indicative of revocation. The latter two methods become effective only when they have been communicated to the attending physician. While such a requirement is obviously necessary, it can become a point of litigation if a physician so acts and a subsequent claim of communication is made by the family, even though there is a degree of protection provided.[56] Also, section 7189.5 appears to provide that for a patient who has signed a directive and then becomes comatose, such directive remains in effect. While this section[57] would seem to have the law err on the side of life (withdrawal of directive without regard to competency), Section 7189.5 appears to reaffirm the patient's right to control his own medical treatment.[58] There is no doubt about the freedom from civil and criminal liability, as well as from a charge of unprofessional conduct. This protection is applied to physicians, health facilities, and licensed health professionals.[59]

While the physician cannot be held liable (civil/criminal) for failing to act upon a directive, he can be held liable for unprofessional conduct for not transferring a patient to a physician who will enact the directive. This reinforces the right to refuse medical treatment.[60] If the patient has not reexecuted a directive, and becomes subsequently qualified to, the physician may gain evidence of the reexecution from the family. This is an issue raised in the Quinlan case. The statute relieves any doubt that such a directive does not constitute suicide, from the standpoint of life insurance and health insurance coverage. Neither can a person be required to sign such a directive to obtain insurance. Section 7194 provides that the execution of a knowingly false directive equals *unlawful* homicide.[61] Finally, and I presume this was to mollify the medical and religious communities, a disaffirmance, of "mercy killing" is provided by the final section of the law.[62]

Except for the State of California, there is no statutory authority for a patient and a physician to enact a "living will." There is, however, case law supported in some aspects by statutory authority that would appear to acknowledge a patient's right to die. It will be interesting to see whether, in the coming years, the California statutory example is followed elsewhere. This area of the law will be affected by the apparent general trend to minimize the involvement of the government in what is appropriately deemed a private decision. It is analogous to the consent section of the Uniform Anatomical Act and to the issue of who has the right to determine what will happen to one's body after death. There the law gives the primary right to the person, with the succeeding classes having no legal basis to interfere with the donation. It is acknowledged that the practical aspects are different.

The right to die, as shown in the California Statute and in the case law cited, is, and will be, predicated on the following: (1) the right of privacy; (2) the right to refuse medical treatment, regardless of who may agree or disagree with the wisdom of such a decision; (3) a changing recognition of the role of the medical professional from that of not only saving lives but also of comforting the dying.

There is another issue that was prominent by its absence—the right (some might say privilege) to have a good quality of life, which is defined as: (1) adequate food, clothing, and shelter; (2) physical and mental health; (3) function in society; (4) access to education; (5)

healthy environment; (6) dignity and self-respect; (7) ability to have responsible use of one's powers.[63]

This highly subjective area probably should be left to the individual decisions and desires of the person. While the right of others to attempt to have another change his mind is considered, it is the individual's ultimate right to reject any such advice as an invasion of privacy, regardless of the source. Where no danger to another nor the creation of a burden to the state exists, there is no basis for intervention.

Religious support was found in several areas, and the most surprising was the brief for the New Jersey Catholic Conference, submitted in the Karen Ann Quinlan case.[64] While their position on euthanasia is most clear, they were emphatic that this was not the question at hand. The following citations are explicative:

[A patient] considered hopeless in the opinion of the competent doctor said that the discontinuance of a respirator as an extraordinary means is not to be considered euthanasia in any way.[65]

This brief lent further support to the traditional role of the doctor as granted by society, but as it is used in conjunction with the consent of the patient. It supported the notion that cessation of *extraordinary* means is allowing "God's intervention" to take its course.[66]

The Jewish view distinguishes between the support of life versus the mitigation of suffering. But such decisions are to be considered only from the moral viewpoint—there is "no punishment by human tribunal."[67] All of this applies to the patient who is suffering from an incurable disease.

The answer to the question at hand is: there is a judicially recognized right to die where such a decision is based on a competent person's right to refuse medical treatment, his right to privacy and that no one else would be "injured." Whether this will gain additional statutory fact beyond California remains to be seen.

Notes

1. Hawaii Legislative Reference Bureau at 2.
2. *Williams*, prologue.

3. *Houts* and *Hauts*, section 1.01 (1).

4. *Id*, at section 1.02 (1).

5. The following definitions from *Black's Law Dictionary* are pertinent:

Death:
The cessation of life; the ceasing to exist; defined by physicians as a total stoppage of the circulation of the blood, and a cessation of the animal and vital functions consequent thereon, such as respiration, pulsation, etc.

Natural death:
A death which occurs by the unassisted operation of natural causes, as distinguished not only from "civil death," but also from "violent death."

Violent death:
One caused or accelerated by the interference of human agency;—distinguished from "natural death."

Euthanasia:
The act or practice of painlessly putting to death persons suffering from incurable and distressing disease. An easy or agreeable death.

Suicide:
Self-destruction; the deliberate termination of one's existence, while in the possession and enjoyment of his mental faculties.

Consent:
A concurrence of wills. Voluntarily yielding the will to the proposition of another; acquiescence or compliance therewith.

6. Kidney transplant programs have developed the use of the term "heart-beating cadaver" to describe the donors for such programs. It is applied to the donor at that point in time when the following events have occurred: family consent for donation is signed, the donor is medically accepted as a donor by the transplant team, and the attending physician has declared the patient dead.

Virtually all such donors are declared dead via the brain death criteria. Hence, the terminology is absolutely descriptive.

7. Hawaii at 2.

8. JAMA 205:337 (1968).

9. See appendix for the University of Miami Criteria of Brain Death.

10. Hawaii at 2. *See also* App. 121 Cal. Rptr. 243 (1975).

11. *Vernon*.

12. *Cohen*.

13. *Houts* and *Hauts*, section 1.01 (2).

14. Hawaii at 2.

15. *Curran* and *Shapiro* at 832.

16. Suicide is the taking of one's own life, and in its technical or legal sense requires that the self-destruction be intentional and by a sane person (83C.J.S.781).

17. See text of The New York Times article.

18. See following section of cases.

19. There is *no* statement regarding euthanasia in C.J.S.

20. Heifetz, ch. 4

21. See Rapouille case to follow and 42 Minn. L. R. 969 (1958).

22. This section is based on *Problems in Hospital Law*, by Aspen Aspen Systems.

23. This section is based on *In the Matter of Karen Ann Quinlan*, which is a compilation of the New Jersey Supreme Court briefs and decision.

24. *Id.* at 302.

25. *Id.* at 306.

26. *Id.* at 313.

27. *Id.* at 315.

28. *Id.* at xvii and 311.

29. *Id.* at 308.

30. *Id.* at xvii.

31. As found in *Curran* and *Shapiro* at 827.

32. All citations are from the case.

33. *Id* at 1681.

34. *Ibid.*

35. *Id.* at 1688.

36. *Id.* at 1689.

37. *Id.* at 1690.

38. *Id.* at 1694.

39. *Id.* at 1701.

40. The proper name is amyotrophic lateral sclerosis. It is "a disease of the motor tracts of the lateral columns of the spinal cord causing progressive muscular atrophy, increasing reflexes, fibrillary twitching, and spastic irritability of the muscles" (*Stedman's Medical Dictionary*, 1961 at 1337).

41. All citations are from the case. There is also an applicable case from Dade County, Civil No. 71-12687 (Dade Co. Cir. Ct., filed July 2, 1971) the court refused to order surgery for a 72-year-old woman where such medical procedures might have prolonged her life, but there was no hope of a cure. Washington Post, July 5, 1971, at 1, column. The Court stated:

Based upon (her) physical condition. . .and the fact that performance of surgery. . .and the administration of further blood transfusions would only result in the painful extension of her life for a short period of time, it is not in the interest of justice for this Court of Equity to order that she be kept alive against her will (Palm Springs Gen. Hosp., Inc. v. Martinez).

42. This section is based on the case cited.

43. *Ibid.*

44. Bergen, at Viii. L. R. 740 (1968), as quoted in the case. This is also similar to the statements in the Hawaiian Legislative study cited herein.

45. The sections are based on the cases cited.

46. 517 F2nd 787 (1975) Poe V. Gerstein.

47. 91 S. Ct. 1848 (1971) Sailer v Leger and Graham v Richardson.

48. 96 S. Ct. 2831 (1976) Planned Parenthood v Danforth.

49. 92 S. Ct. 1029 (1972) Eisenstadt v Baird.

50. California Statutes, Chapter 3.9, Sections 7185 to 7195.

51. *Id.* at Section 7187.

52. *Id.* at Section 7188.

53. For the patient in a nursing home, there is a separate section (7188.5) that places additional requirements to make the directive effective. The basis for this is given as the fact that some patients "may be so insulated from a voluntary decisionmaking role. . . ."

54. This is consistent with 201 A2nd 537 (1964).

55. California Statutes, Section 1789.

56. *Id.* at Section 7189:
(b) There shall be no criminal or civil liability on the part of any person for failure to act upon a revocation made pursuant to this section unless that person has actual knowledge of the revocation.

57. *Ibid.*

58. The consent section (2) from the Florida Uniform Anatomical Gift Act should be noted:
    (a) Any individual of sound mind and 18 years of age or more may give all or any part of his body for any purpose specified in section 3, the gift to take effect upon death.
    (b) Any of the following persons, in order of priority stated, when persons in prior classes are not available at the time of death, and in the absence of actual notice of contrary indications by the decedent or actual notice of opposition by a member of the same or prior class, may give all or any part of the decedent's body for any purpose specified in section 3:
        1. the spouse,
        2. an adult son or daughter,
        3. either parent,
        4. an adult brother or sister,
        5. a guardian of the person of the decedent at the time of his death,
        6. any other person authorized or under obligation to dispose of the body.
provided, however, no gift shall be made by the spouse if any adult son or daughter shall object thereto (Florida Statutes 736.20 - 31).

59. California Statutes, Section 7190.

60. *Id*. at Section 7191.

61. *Id*. at Section 7192.

62. *Id*. at Section 7195.

63. Hill and Wang, ch. 5.

64. *In the Matter of Karen Ann Quinlan* at 198ff.

65. *Id*. at 199.

66. *Id*. at 200, quoting Pope Pius XII to the International Congress of Anesthesiologists, November 24, 1957.

67. 31 N.Y.U. L.R. 1160 at 1203f.

References

Aries, P. 1976. *Western Attitudes Towards Death*. Baltimore, Maryland: Johns Hopkins University Press.

Black, H. C. 1968. *Black's Law Dictionary*, ed. 4 St. Paul, Minnesota: West Publishing Co.

Cohen, B. D. 1976. *Karen Ann Quinlan*. New York: Nash Publishing Co.

Curran, W. J. and D. Shapiro. 1970. *Law Medicine and Forensic Sciences*, 2nd ed. Boston: Little Brown and Co.

Heifetz, M. and C. Mongel. 1975. *The Right to Die*. New York: G. P. Putnam and Sons.

Houts, M. and I. Hauts. 1978. *Courtroom Medicine*, vols. 3, 3A, 3B. New York: Matthew Bender.

Humber, J. M. and R. F. Almedes. 1976. *Biomedical Ethics and the Law*. New York: Plenum Press.

Krantz, M. J. 1974. *Dying and Dignity*. Springfield, Illinois: Charles C. Thomas.

Ludes, F. J. and H. J. Gilbert. 1963. *Sociology of Death*. New York: American Law Book Co.

Vernon, G. M. 1970. *Sociology of Death*. New York: Ronald Press.

Williams, R. H. 1973. *To Live and to Die: When, Why and How*. New York: Springer Verlag.

In the Matter of Karen Ann Quinlan, 1976. Vol. 2. Washington, D. C.: University Publications of America.

Problems in Hospital Law. 1974. 2nd ed. Rockville, Maryland: Aspen Systems Corp.

Towards a Definition of Death. 1977. Hawaii: Legislative Reference Bureau.

Who Shall Live? Man's Control Over Birth and Death, A Report for the American Friends Service Committee. 1970. New York: Hill and Wang.

74   Richard A. Metz

Primary Listing of Cases

Erickson v. Dilgard, 252 NYS2nd 705-6 (1962).

In re Green, 292 A2nd 387 (1971).

Fontenot v. Southern Farm Bureau Insurance, 304 SO2nd 690 (1975).

People v. Roberts, 178 NW 690 (1920).

Raleigh Fitkin-Paul Morgan Hospital v. Anderson, 201 A2nd 537 (1964).

133 NE 567 (1921).

Woods v. Lancet, 102 NE2nd 691 (1951).

United States v. Francios, 164 F2nd 163 (1947).

Application of President and Directors of Georgetown College, 331 F2nd 1000 (1963).

Belchertown v. Saikewicz, 370 NE2nd 417 (1977).

In re Brooks' Estate, 205 NE2nd 435 (1965).

Consent re: Surgical Operation, 76 ALR 562-9.

Compulsory Medical Care for Adult, 9 ALR3rd 1391-8.

State of Calif v. Saldana, App 121 Cal. Rptr 243 (1975).

Strunk v. Strunk, 445 SW2nd 145 (1969).

The Florida Law Weekly 1978, Case #78-1486, 1273-74, Satz v. Perlmutter.

Griswold v. State of Connecticut, 85 SCT 1678 (1965).

Eisenstadt v. Baird, 92 SCT 1029 (1972).

Planned Parenthood v. Danforth, 96 SCT 2831 (1976).

Cleveland Board of Ed. v. LaFleur; Cohen v. Chesterfield Co. Sch. Bd., 94 SCT 791.

Sailer v. Leger; Graham v. Richardson, 91 SCT 1848 (1971).

Stradley v. Anderson, 478 F2nd 188 (1973).

Scott v. Plante, 532 F2nd 939.

Poe v. Gerstein, 517 F2nd 787 (1975).

Law Reviews

30 Ohio State Law Journal 32.

12 San Diego Law Review 424.

22 University of Florida Law Review 368 (1970).

27 Baylor Law Review 62.

42 Minnesota Law Review 969 (1958).

27 Baylor Law Review 62, 67.

30 Ohio State Law Journal 32, 51 (1969).
57 California Law Review 671 (1969).
21 Vanderbilt Law Review 352 (1968).
118 New York Law Journal 486 (1968).
31 NYU Law Review 1160 (1956).
42 Minnesota Law Review 969 (1958).
43 Minnesota Law Review 1 (1958).
15 Southwest Law Journal 393.
21 University of Florida Law Review 452/22-368.
54 ABAJ 855
31 Ohio State Law Journal 66, 96.

Other

California Statutes Section 7185, Health Code.
Journal of the American Medical Association (JAMA), American Medical Association, Chicago, Illinois.

Appendix

UNIVERSITY OF MIAMI
Criteria of Brain Death

With the advent of cardiopulmonary resuscitation and the transplantation of vital organs, the determination of neurological death has received renewed attention by medical, legal, and religious authorities. The following criteria of brain death have been established by the University of Miami Transplant Committee, March 1973:

1. Absence of spontaneous movement and response to stimulation.
2. Absence of spontaneous respiration.
3. Absence of brain stem reflexes.
4. Potentially reversible etiology, i.e., barbiturates, hypothermia, and/or age under 12 years, must all be considered prior to finally diagnosing brain death.
5. Isoelectric electroencephalogram is required when available at time of evaluation of potential donor.

6. Repeat evaluation including EEG (when available) should be performed after 24 hours, when the condition of potential donor allows this time lapse.
7. If severe structural brain damage is found, which is incompatible with brain function, brain death can be declared without the previous criteria.
8. Declaration of brain death must be made and recorded by the patient's primary physician and by a neurologist or neurosurgeon not directly involved in the care of the patient.

7

Humanistic Care of the Dying

David W. Moller

The final medical solution to human problems: remove everything from the body that is diseased or protesting, leaving only enough organs which by themselves, or hooked up to appropriate machines—still justify calling what is left of a person a "case"; and call the procedure "humanectomy."—T. Szasz. 1974. *The Second Sin* (New York: Doubleday)

A hospital is a bureaucratically organized *gesellschaft* type of social institution whose function is to treat and heal disease. The task of healing is primarily pursued and accomplished vis-a-vis scientific, rational methods. According to the medical point of view, rationalization, standardization, and depersonalization are "worth the price" when medical results benefit the patient. The underlying premise of this orientation is that the vital needs of man are purely technical. The requirements of a patient's humanity, therefore, yield wholly to some means of formal-technical analysis that can be carried out by specialists possessing certain impenetrable skills that can translate patient needs into a series of management procedures and regimens. If a problem does not have an objective base and a technical solution, it must not be a real problem worthy of real attention.

This purely scientific base of American medicine subjugates the patient in a straitjacket of rational fervor and emotional neglect. The injustices of the rational approach to patient management develop directly from the denial or obliteration of human concerns and needs. The task of this paper, then, is to explore from a sociological point of view the hospital as a structure of dehumanization for the medical patient in general and the dying person in particular. Suggestions are made regarding a humanistic model of care for those dying within the institutional strictures of a bureaucratic social structure.

The Hospital as Total Social Institution

Every social institution is capable of dominating the time, interests, and activities of individuals in them. Some do so to a greater degree than others. A total institution is total in this dominating capacity and is generally characterized by physical separation from and blocking of social intercourse with the outside world.[1] A hospital possesses this general separational dominating dimension while being specifically designed to treat those individuals who are incapable of self-care and who are no real threat to society.[2] To be sure, this is one feature that distinguishes the hospital from other total institutions such as prisons or monasteries.

The total institutional establishment, while representing the most efficient form of social organization, is one that is also quite morally suspect. Specifically, a total institution mortifies an individual's self-concept and violates an individual's personal dignity. A hospital "accomplishes" this through a variety of means, several of which are considered here.

The initiation ritual of admission marks the first curtailment of individual identity. The person who walks into the admissions office to be admitted is wheeled out as a patient. A process of role disengagement, henceforth, begins. The person is being redefined into a patient who will be treated by the hospital not in terms of personal worth but by nonhuman medical considerations.[3] The initial moments of socialization in the hospital ward further substantiate self-mortification. The staff "welcome" the admission with a barrage of directives and questions that give the new admission a clear understanding that he/she will be treated from a nonpersonal medical viewpoint. Newly admitted patients also begin to recognize at this point that deference and obedience are expected of them as they relate to physicians and nurses. Personal identity becomes largely extinguished when personal clothing is stripped away and the patient is dressed in hospital garb. More specifically, as the individual is stripped of his usual appearance and of the equipment and services by which he maintains it, the result is a suffering of personal defacement. This loss of what has been termed "identity kit," prevents the patient from presenting his usual image of himself to others.[4]

The transfiguration from person to patient results in a process of dehumanization to the extent that the hospital staff loses sight of the subjective dimensions of an individual and focuses largely or exclusively on objective, technical concerns. This objectification of personhood is functional from the medical point of view, for a person's body can be examined, probed, poked, and explored more readily if the concern is merely one of isolating and treating a specific disease. To be sure, a violation of the territories of the self becomes especially difficult if that self is defined in terms of personal, subjective criteria. Thus, the total social institution of the hospital diminishes the social self of an individual by treating him as a "nonperson" medical entity. Erving Goffman eloquently describes this process as:

...the wonderful brand of "nonperson" treatment found in the medical world, whereby the patient is greeted with what passes as civility and said farewell to in the same fashion, with everything in between going on as if the patient weren't there as a social person at all, but only as a possession someone has left behind.[5]

The essential point to be made is that there is a fundamental dilemma between a people orientation and an object orientation in the institutional treatment of the ill. The conflict is essentially one of humane standards versus institutional efficiency. Owing to the rational foundation of the contemporary hospital, the subjectivity of working with such people is often deferred in preference to treating patients *objectively* and *rationally* by *professionals* on the basis of *information* technically collected. As Henry Heinemann notes:

Since the introduction of modern technology, the hospital has lost its aura of being a place of comfort and has instead become an establishment resembling a factory, where illnesses are taken care of rather than human beings.[6]

Patient Alienation Within the Hospital

Patients within hospitals have become prisoners—of rationality, technical orientation, and total institutional dominance. In this sense a hospital is a manipulative institution[7] in that it primarily serves its own philosophy and orientation of bureaucratic rationality in its everyday workings. Loss of personal identity and dignity is often the price paid for medical efficiency. To the extent to which this price is paid, individual patients become alienated within the hospital setting.

Alienation as a concept presently and traditionally has held a central place in sociological study of society. Indeed, at the present time, in all the social sciences, the various symptoms of alienation have a foremost place in studies of human relations. Investigations of the "unattached," the "marginal," the "obsessive," the "normless," and the isolated individual all testify to the central place occupied by the hypothesis of alienation in contemporary social science.[8] It needs to be immediately recognized, however, that alienation as a concept abounds in the sociological literature only to the extent that alienation as a social reality characterizes everyday life.

Alienation has been variously defined by social scientists as referring to that process which separates man from necessary and inherent characteristics of the human species. A variety of measures of alienation have been advanced, three of which are considered in terms of general dimensions and their specific application to dying people in a hospital setting.

Powerlessness,[9] or the impossibility context, refers to the belief of an individual that he cannot determine or influence a desired goal. The feeling that "there is not much I can do about the significant personal and social problems confronting me" is a typical illustration of the powerlessness dimension of alienation. The feeling of being powerless may be the consequence of "natural"[10] or "artificial" causes, that is to say, it may be in the nature of being human to be unable to do something about a specific problem, or such personal impotence may be imposed on individuals by society and social structure.

Death is an inherent feature of life. In the final analysis, despite medical triumphs, it is a future natural dimension that man cannot defeat. Hence, powerlessness in the face of death is intrinsic to the human experience. From a social perspective, powerlessness abounds for the dying individual. Is it really conceivable for a dying person, a dying patient who has had personal identity stripped away, to be able to affect decisions regarding even his own fate in a meaningful way? Powerlessness is, therefore, a social construction of the nonperson treatment imposed upon dying individuals in the total institution of the hospital. So total is the suppressing of a dying patient's personal presence that his fate can be openly discussed around his bed by a variety of experts without the discussants' having to feel undue concern. A technical vocabulary presumably unknown to the patient helps in this regard.[11] Thus, the castration of personal identity and power very deeply and uniquely frustrates individuals in directly determining important sociopersonal issues during their dying days.

A second indicator of alienation is social isolation,[12] the feeling of being without social support and social assistance. This leaves us feeling anxious, vulnerable, alone, and lonely. While loneliness may be a condition inherent to the human experience, social science has effectively demonstrated that as society has progressed, becoming more "advanced" and scientized, loneliness correspondingly has burgeoned. Among the themes of our best present-day drama and art are conceptions of fragmentation, suffering, and despair. Contemporary literature is dominated by themes of loneliness, disillusionment, misunderstanding, and disaffection. In short, life American style is characterized by social polarization, and the drift of our times is away from solidarity, fellowship, and dialogue.[13]

The social isolation of the dying is a reflection of the physical structure, the philosophy, the norms, and the rules and regulations of the total institution of death. I have noted elsewhere[14] that interpersonal fellowship and support are rare "commodities" at the deathbed today. Patients die without the emotional support of people. Present are the experts who focus on the technical aspects of the process and professional equipment functionally carrying out their mandates. It has been documented that the staff of the total institutional hospital, namely, physicians and nurses, neglect their patients when medical intervention is no longer feasible or effective. Specifically, it has been shown that physicians tend to avoid dying patients, and nurses respond more slowly to the signal calls of the terminally ill than to those not dying.[15] Friends and relatives are but minimally integrated into the everyday happenings and experiences of the institutionalized dying patient. In short, social isolation is a normative sociostructural feature of the way people die in America today.

A third indicator of alienation is species estrangement.[16] To be human is to directly engage in relationships with and influence and shape one's social environment. It has been argued that the capacity of being in control of our lives and environments is the first and last ethical word of being human.[17] Indeed, our nonhuman animal counterparts are required to adapt to their environments, whereas man is able to shape and control his environment. The most simplistic illustration is that, while a bear hibernates for the winter, man builds shelter and designs heaters to provide warmth. Hence, animals adapt to and men confront, shape, and determine their environments to a large degree. Therefore, self-determination and social control are distinctively human characteristics, and if we become estranged from self-determination and control, we likewise become alienated from what makes us human.

The nonperson treatment of the dying medical patient is a prototypical example of species estrangement. The subjectivity of personhood is rendered powerless as the dying person becomes reduced to a mere assemblage of objective parts to be treated by medical techniques. As human subjectivity is denied in preference to patient objectification, species estrangement emerges. Subjects are actors in control, whereas objects are acted upon. The extent to which a dying person's subjectivity, his personhood, is denied by technical medical intervention is the extent to which he cannot be in self-determining control of his own physiological and social lives. This theme finds expression in the inimitable words of Ivan Illich:

The chief function of the physician becomes that of umpire. He is the agent, a representative of the social body, with the duty to make sure that everyone plays the game according to the rules. The rules, of course, forbid leaving the game and dying in any fashion which has not been specified by the umpire. Death no longer occurs except as the self fulfilling prophecy of the medicine man.[18]

Death, the final life process of the dying individual, is henceforth determined and controlled not by the individual but by his medical experts.

Powerlessness, social isolation, and species estrangement are three measures of alienation that beleaguer the dying patient. They are a direct development of the nonperson treatment inherent in a total social institution. As the indicators increase, so will patient alienation. As powerlessness increases, alienation increases. However, as powerlessness, social isolation, and species estrangement increase together, alienation increases to an even greater degree. This appears to be the case in the medical treatment of the dying. The problem of alienation, therefore, becomes a major issue that needs to be addressed in any consideration of the human dimensions of care for the critically ill person.

A Blueprint of a Sociomedical Structure for the Terminally Ill

A critical care facility, whether it be called hospice or otherwise, should seek to reconcile the apparently opposing forces of medical efficiency with humanistic concern. Promoting the maximum quality of human life feasible should be the goal of the facility. Attempts should be consciously made to minimize the alienating and dehumanizing consequences of the total institution. Personhood should be the sine qua non of the philosophy of care.

It is precisely in this spirit that a social blueprint has been developed. This should be seen merely as a preliminary attempt to actively combat the problem of alienation previously discussed. The proposal is divided into three distinct but interrelated areas: the initiation, the staff, and the support mechanisms.

The Initiation

1. The initial "welcome" into the facility should be made by nonmedical personnel—social psychologist, social worker, clergy. This will serve the vital function of assuring the individual that his personhood is of central concern.

2. The individual should not be stripped of personal possessions and clothing. A set of day and night clothes should be encouraged.

Personal choice of clothing will help to preserve the individual's social self and will allow for the individual to decide what image to present to others.

3. Individuals should be encouraged to bring their own bed clothes (sheets, pillowcases, blankets, etc.). This will help to personalize the institutional environment with a touch of warmth.

4. New admissions should be introduced to other individuals on their wing and to the facility staff. This will generate a sense of interpersonal familiarity for the newcomer.

5. Psychosocial biographies should be obtained on each individual and be required reading for all staff. The biographies will provide reassurance of the centrality of personhood to the care being offered and will also generate an invaluable source of relevant personal and social information on each person.

The Staff

1. Physicians and nurses should undergo a thanatology sensitization course. It has been widely noted that health care personnel have been ineffectually trained to deal with the human dimension of medical care. It is therefore essential to formally counterbalance the pure scientism and rigorous objectivity of medical training with a course rich in social science and humanities underpinnings.

2. The use of objectifying language should be discouraged. Person or individual is certainly more desirable than patient or case. The important function of the linguistic concern is to motivate the professional staff to view people from a personal, as well as medical, perspective.

3. Nurses should be dressed in comfortable, functional, "nonuniformed" clothing. Physicians should be discouraged from wearing white coats. This will enable people to begin to see medical staff as more than technical experts.

4. All major medical decisions should be discussed by the individual, his physician, and another staff member of the person's choice. A family representative may, upon request, be included in the discussions. Final decision-making responsibility should reside with the individual. Choices made as freely as possible will help to minimize the controlling

power of the medical profession, increasing personal autonomy and self-determination.

5. A psychosocial consultation board should be established. This board will meet on regular occasions to discuss relevant issues of each case and make relevant suggestions about caregiving. This board should be composed of medical and nonmedical personnel.

6. A professional support group should be established to meet on a regular basis to discuss issues of concern to the staff. This group will provide a formal network of support for staff working in an emotionally difficult and draining area.

Support Systems

1. Psychosocial support and therapy should be available for the individual and his family. The presence of psychosocial professional support will assist them in coping with the emotional pain and suffering of the dying process.

2. The facility should possess a reasonable religious orientation. Religious faith and practice can be an enormous source of solace and comfort in facing the terror of death. Spirituality should therefore be integrated into the philosophy and workings of the structure.

3. A "community" meeting room should be available. All individuals should have input into determining the nature and role of community activities (lectures, films, minicourses, discussions.). The planning of a variety of activities will serve to integrate meaning into the daily schedule of participating individuals.

4. Visiting hours should be open on a 24-hour basis. It is not important for visitors to be constantly present, but such a visiting schedule assures people that family and other loved ones can be present if the need arises.

5. A community dining facility will serve to humanize the facility. One of the major distinguishing human characteristics is that, while animals feed for sustenance, humans dine. Providing a facility whereby the community can dine by themselves or with staff or family can generate a vital humanizing network of support.

6. Continuing bereavement support and services should be offered to the family during the funeral and postfuneral mourning period. The

extent to which this proposal is successful will indicate the general success of the facility in integrating family, staff, and dying individuals into a collective, caring community.

Conclusion

It needs to be stressed that death is not the dignifying, joyful event that some theorists would lead us to believe it is. The process of dying is inherently terrifying and frightening, and present-day medicinal treatment of the dying exacerbates the indignities of the experience. This recognition should be the point of departure for a critical care facility: seeking to design a structure sufficiently rich with sincere social and human caring so as to begin to minimize the indignities currently associated with death American style.

Notes

1. E. Goffman, 1961. *Asylums*. New York: Doubleday, ch. 1.)

2. *Ibid.*

3. M. Krant, 1972. "In the Context of Dying." In B. Schoenberg, et al., eds. *Psychosocial Aspects of Terminal Care*. New York: Columbia University Press, pp. 201-9.

4. K. Kesey, 1965. *One Flew Over the Cuckoo's Nest*. New York: Signet.

5. Goffman, *Asylums,* p. 315.

6. H. Heinemann, 1972. "Human Values in the Medical Care of the Terminally Ill." In Schoenberg et al., eds., *Psychosocial Aspects,* p.22.

7. I. Illich, 1973. *Tools for Convivality*. New York: Harper and Row.

8. R. Nisbet, 1953. *The Quest for Community*. New York: Oxford University Press, p. 15.

9. M. Seeman, 1959. "On the Meaning of Alienation." *American Sociological Review* (October) 24: 83-91.

10. T. O'Dea, 1966. *The Sociology of Religion*. Englewood Cliffs, N.J.: Prentice-Hall, ch. 1.

11. Goffman, *Asylums*, p. 315.

12. Seeman, "Alienation."

13. K. Kenniston, 1965. *The Uncommitted*. New York: Harcourt, Brace, Jovanovitch, p. 4.

14. D. W. Moller, 1980. "Dying and Fellowship." Presentation at Foundation of Thanatology Symposium, Bethlehem, Pennsylvania.

15. B. Glasser and A. Strauss. 1965. *Awareness of Dying*. Chicago: Aldine.

16. K. Marx. 1964. *Early Writings*. (Edited by T. B. Bottomore). New York: McGraw Hill.

17. E. Fromm, 1976. *To Have Or To Be*. New York: Bantam Press.

18. I. Illich, 1976. *Medical Nemesis*. New York: Pantheon, p. 285.

8

Death with Dignity

William Regelson

As a cancer specialist for more than 25 years, I have seen the suffering that dying causes and I understand the concern that has led sincere people to propose right to die statutes. But I also see missing from both the national debate and the various attempts at a legal resolution a careful consideration of the way these proposals would change the role of the physician in American society. Whether ignored or unconsidered, the implications of death with dignity are many and complicated. They must be examined before any decisions are reached or the result will be dangerous legal precedents and simplifications.

All of the proposed Death with Dignity bills have the same stamp of concern for the rights of the dying, but what actually underlies the whole issue are the fright and embarrassment of the living. We are afraid, not just of dying, but of the way we will die. No longer embarrassed by the facts of life, we are now ashamed of the facts of death: the bedpan, the catheter, and the respirator. In an age when technology can destroy mankind, there is also an understandable fear of the potential tyranny of machines, even those created to prolong life. We want to return to a simpler way of dying. We want a classical, clean, convenient death.

Proposed Death with Dignity laws may be primarily based on motives of kindness and sympathy but, as sold by their advocates, they constitute a psychological, social, and economic laundering of a dirty process. With their own vision of the horrors of prolonged debilitation and dying, they establish their own truth, publicize their "good death," and seek to legislate it. The motives may be sincere, but what matters is the result—a statutory change in our view of those most dependent on society. The patients most often involved in these considerations are not the acutely ill but the chronically ill and the helpless. And I am concerned about those of us who play a role in their care, the physicians who are now the arbiters of their death. Before we can reach a rational and kind solution, we must have a clear and factual view of the problem. Unfortunately, even the most vocal advocates of death with dignity seem to lack such a view. If a general familiarity with life support systems existed, perhaps the melodramatic image of tubes and pumps and the vague fear of medicine's technical advances would disappear.

Some of the most commonly used life support techniques are intravenous or tube feedings that sustain life through hydration. These are used in advanced diseases when the patient is unable to maintain an adequate fluid intake. Physicians use these infusions even when they recognize the imminence of death, because without them the patient would die of dehydration—or in simpler, harsher terms, he would die of thirst. To deny a patient this treatment would be the equivalent of leaving him to die under a desert sun. Such support is an act of kindness, even if it prolongs life only for a few hours. Who can know how much awareness and pain an individual feels when he is in a coma or semicoma and cannot communicate? Parenteral fluid support has been discontinued to let death take over, but only in clearly irreversible cases of very deep coma and shock.

Similarly, nasal oxygen is used to remove the sense of oppression and suffocation that patients who are deprived of effective lung space or blood volume feel. Some physicians may continue to use oxygen for long periods, but in no way would it keep a terminal patient alive for days. It is a simple supportive measure that can be removed.

Artificial pacemakers, in widespread use for several years, are the best example of medical technology that prolongs human life. They allow the patient to return to a fairly normal, and in some cases vigorous, life. In the intensive care and coronary care units, the pacemaker saves lives. If we do not venture the use of such instruments to maintain effective heartbeat, what kind of gains to normal survival can we expect? Though most right-to-die advocates do not oppose the pacemaker's use, their fear of medical machinery, if made into law, could end the use and development of similar devices.

Blood transfusions have also long been used by physicians to sustain and prolong the patient's life. Where one draws the line and decides to stop transfusions for obviously terminal patients is a difficult decision to make. Even if one knows the futility of continuing, it is hard to order a cessation when a patient requests more blood. When the patient is in shock or coma, the decision is easier.

Some of the most common grotesque images of life support systems are projected by the feeding or drainage tubes attached to the patient. Tubes may be uncomfortable, but a distended gut accompanied by cramping and nausea causes more pain than any tube. The same is true for a distended bladder: try to hold in your urine beyond a critical time, and you will know what distention is like. Tubes relieve distention, but at what point does one remove the tube? Should one instead increase the level of narcotics and make the use of tubes incidental?

A recently developed life support procedure is "hyperalimentation," which provides intravenous nourishment in liquid form sufficient to sustain life in the absence of oral intake and bowel functions for weeks and months. Hyperalimentation can save the lives of severe burn victims or patients with bowel destruction or fistulas from ileitis, colitis, blood clots, or trauma. If one fails in attempting this procedure and the patient dies, it is always possible for someone to say that one kept the individual alive inappropriately, but no physician would use this procedure with all its cost and effort unless there was some hope for decent life.

The mechanical respirator has received the most attention in recent media coverage of the death with dignity issue, with particular reference to the Quinlan case. Two kinds of respirators exist: the first aids voluntary breathing and coughing to clear the lungs of secretion and adjust blood gases to normal levels. It is most often used in postoperative patients or in emphysema and bronchiectasis patients who need help in getting rid of secretions. The second is the full-assist or positive-pressure respirator, which completely takes over a patient's damaged or nonfunctioning respiratory system. Contrary to popular conception, however, these full assist machines are rarely used.

Of the 29,000 patients admitted to the Medical College of Virginia (Richmond) in 1974, only 440 used this machine for an average of only 2.54 days, with time on the machine ranging from several hours to 44 days. We have analyzed the use of this machine in a random selection of 50 patients. There was no case of these respirators being used where an acute situation could not be remedied, except after brain death when the patient's respiration was sustained for organ transplant purposes with the family's approval. Once the machine was used, there was no fear of stopping its use on the part of any physician, despite the fact that it would result in the physician's responsibility for the legal and medical brain death of the patient. There were no horror stories of machine-driven living dead, only the practical mechanics of sustaining living people through periods of crisis that might mean decent survival.

In 1970, Dr. James Bartlet, Medical Director of Strong Memorial Hospital in Rochester, New York, conducted a survey into the use of resuscitation for terminal patients. Dr. Bartlet studied 100 consecutive deaths out of the 772 patients who had died in his hospital. In 79 of those 100 cases, death was anticipated by the physicians. In the 21 cases where death was not anticipated, 17 received either respiratory assist and/or cardiac massage. Two of those 17 had emergency surgery; one had an artificial pacemaker installed.

Of the 79 patients whose deaths were expected, 21 had cancer, and no attempts at resuscitation were made. Several of the cancer patients were on oxygen or intravenous support; one was on an ice blanket. Another 27 of the anticipated death cases suffered from heart or lung diseases; six had assorted trauma, or kidney or liver failure. Of this group, 11 were on life support machines. Six patients died of vascular occlusion or stroke. In only seven of the 79 cases were attempts at emergency resuscitation made in spite of the severity of the illness and the poor prognosis. Only two survived resuscitation, and they died shortly afterward.

Summary statistics from the Rochester experience show that only 15 percent of the deaths occurred during prolonged hospitalization, and 50 percent of those who died had recent previous stays in the hospital.

From an examination of these figures, one is hard pressed to find a problem that could be solved by legislation. We can only hope that right-to-die advocates would not find fault with heroic lifesaving measures in the 17 of 21 in whom death was not expected.

After-the-fact analysis shows that the attempted resuscitations of the seven patients who were expected to die were errors. But it should be obvious that physicians have to react swiftly and instinctively to medical emergencies, and sometimes the situation is ambiguous. The fact that no advanced cancer patients were resuscitated in the Rochester study is important. The cardiac, renal, and severely traumatized patients who did receive these emergency efforts can sometimes survive at levels of comfort despite chronic injury. Here lay the ambiguity that led to heroic but futile measures.

In my cancer chemotherapy unit, the nurses and housestaff exercise good judgment, and each case is discussed in detail as to the emergency life support methods that should and should not be used. However, if sudden and unexplained complications developed in a patient whose prognosis was probable death, I would not hesitate to try to save him, provided I thought that radiotherapy or chemotherapy could produce a decent survival.

None of these life support measures as used in most general hospitals refers to the crux of the problem for euthanasia or death with dignity advocates. The real issue for them is, not the hospital's dealing with acute medical situations, but the chronic care facilities such as nursing homes and mental institutions where the old and chronically ill go to die and frequently take their time about it. The problem involves those patients who are severely handicapped, be it from mental retardation, birth defects, trauma, senility, stroke, or an advanced cancer.

Life support systems are often necessary for patients in coma, but it should be made clear that not all comatose patients are terminal. At one time, years ago, they were. But with all the developments in medical technology, those suffering from diabetes, ventricular fibrillation, renal failure, and coronary shock can survive. Unless there is a flat electro-encephalogram, brain recovery is possible. To refer to the celebrated Karen Quinlan case, she *does* have a measurable brain wave. Even if her chances of recovery are one in a thousand, should she be denied that chance by the removal of the supportive systems? The physician's proper role is as the affirmer of life. He should never be made its denier by law, which is what proposed death with dignity bills would do.

The potential problems raised by House Bill 620 are worse than the one it proposes to cure. In attempting to simplify the problem of death for patient, family, and physician, the bill only complicates it with legal documents whose validity must be checked and rechecked. When the emergency medical decisions of life and death arise, there is no time to check the elaborate legal status of wills. Who will determine the timing of the plug pulling, the dictates of the living will or the physician? Suppose the terminal, comatose patient, while having dictated the time of his death, had neglected to indicate whether his organs could be transplanted to other needy, desperate patients. Could the physician artificially sustain his life until transplant approval from the relatives had been obtained, or must the plug be pulled immediately and thus destroy any possibilities of transplant? Only another addendum to the right-to-die statute could decide, and the same would be true of many other medical questions. Problems that can now be solved by personal judgment of the physician could be solved only be the further complicated and prolonged involvement of legislatures and courts. Such bills establish only a new bureaucracy of death, and despite the intended advantages the response can only be—who needs it?

The key to all euthanasia bills relates to definitions and decisions made by physicians. The bill begins with an effort to define legally the concept of terminality. The prognosis about whether a patient's illness or injury is terminal is a difficult one even in medical terms; legal efforts to define it only further becloud the issue.

The number of diseases formerly thought to be incurable and terminal that have now become treatable must be remembered. Formerly, Parkinson's disease was considered an untreatable manifestation of viral or vascular damage to a brain center. But now we have discovered that it is a biochemical disease related to the brain's copper levels that can be modified by dopamine. For similar examples, one needs only to look at acute lymphocytic leukemia in children and Hodgkin's disease. Five or ten years ago, individuals with these diseases had limited survival rates; today they can be cured, and other forms of leukemia and lymphoma are also now responding to treatment. Osteogenic sarcoma can now be treated, and a prolongation of decent survival is currently seen in a wide range of tumors, including myeloma and those of the breast, prostate, testicles, and even of the bowel.

Similar statements can easily and triumphantly be made about most infectious diseases, certain aspects of renal disease, and of course, diabetes. What will we discover for other presently "terminal" diseases in the future? What will we think of and do for senility in the years to come? To quit the struggle, to resign oneself to death because of present and codified definitions of terminality, because of a patient's debility and depression, is contrary to the physician's role as healer.

In my practice, I have seen definitions of "terminal" deny a patient effective treatment because it would prolong his life only for three to six months rather than produce a "cure." Yet the experience and quality of life in those last months is valid and extremely meaningful for the person who is ill. We must realize that new ideas can change the character of illness and improve the quality of life. We must start from a base of optimism and be permitted to pull the plug only as a last resort and let only brain death beyond our control enter. Medical students, physicians, nurses, and all of us involved in primary care must not renege on our commitment to the chronically ill, the debilitated, and the helpless. Yet, right-to-die legislation makes such an abnegation not only permissible but also easier to quit supporting a patient because it will become a legal passport for convenience over responsibility. Although advocates deny it, right-to-die legislation is euthanasia legislation because the implication is there that, given the lawyer's certification on the living will, the plug can be pulled without legal vulnerability.

Death with dignity may become death as convenience. With a legal permission and emphasis on "the good death" of euthanasia, rather than wait for a possible cure or decent interval of survival, the physician and family might choose the easier road and let the patient die to avoid causing pain and inconvenience to the relatives. With the heavy costs of medical care, it would certainly be financially convenient to pull the plug. Would euthanasia then be equally applied to rich and poor? Will it be free of economic and social pressures? Will today's legislation of the free choice of one's right to die become an *insistence* that the terminally ill exercise that right? What of those who signed no living will and have no relatives to sign one for them? Who will guarantee their "rights?" The state? The hospital administration, looking for any means to cut constantly increasing deficits? Remember, when one takes the legalized euthanasia step for the first time, it becomes easier on each subsequent occasion. Society's attitudes are not immutable. Abortion, once strictly illegal and generally considered immoral and akin to murder, is now a popularly accepted, easily obtained operation, and the unwanted unborn are discarded like beer cans along the highway. Euthanasia does not deal with an apersonal fetus; it concerns a basic safeguard in our society— the fundamental role of the physician and his or her attitude toward human life.

Doctors withdraw life support now without the stigma of committing murder and without the need to codify or be protected by special laws. The reason why this can be done is based on the fact that the doctor is being judged by peers: colleagues, nurses, housestaff, pharmacists, the family, and others who are part of the support system that sustains the patient. We have to ask the question—will right-to-die legislation change the system or improve what we have?

It should not be easy for us to let the sick die; we must hold to our image as advocates for life. Passive euthanasia should be looked upon as failure, not as an act of kindness, for to give it priority will make it easy to let those die who may have options that include decent survival. Legislation adds another layer to the complicated matrix of law. It puts a lawyer into the picture, but does it give us anything in return? It alters the balance of moral responsibility in the same way that legalized gambling, prostitution, and drinking change the pattern of use for what is available. In these cases, the choice affects only the individual who makes it. In the case of the legalized living will, the choice is made for the individual by others no matter what the intent of the individual who signs the living will. The result of making withdrawal of life support a legally sanctioned event is to change the priority of its use, but the indulgence is more potent than a thin wallet or a hangover or a case of venereal disease.

The death with dignity bills will create unneeded and ill-considered changes that may result in an irrevocable turnabout in America's medical traditions. The issue does need to be clarified but not statutorily oversimplified.

9

Patient Rights and Responsibilities in Irreversible Disease

Ruth D. Abrams

The concept of individual patient rights is welcomed by the majority of people. Yet what we first considered a victory we soon find to be as much of a burden as a blessing. In no other area of life does taking responsibility produce more satisfaction and at the same time more personal hardship than in the preterminal and terminal stages of irreversible disease. The patient's responsibilities loom very large and produce a new hardship for the physician—the invasion of privacy, which has for too long been protected by the profession. This presentation focuses on the patient with breast cancer in the preterminal and terminal stages.

My experience has been in the cancer field—as a counselor in many clinic settings; in research at the Massachusetts General Hospital and at Harvard's Laboratory of Community Psychiatry, and in private practice with patients who live and die with cancer. Much of what follows applies to patients with any irreversible disease who face dying and death.

• The patient's first right is to be told her diagnosis and probable prognosis by the physician in charge—but *only* if she wants it. Donald S. Kornfeld, addressing this issue in the *Cancer Journal for Clinicians* (January 1977) wrote:

To assume, even were the truth known, that all patients want that kind of truth or would benefit from it is a dangerous generalization. I have spoken to many patients who have been told "the truth" and have chosen to deny it. I have known others who have been told "the truth" and become depressed or anxious to the point where their last days, months or years were spent in terror of death. And, of course, there were those who have heard "the truth" and benefitted from this knowledge, living out their days the better for having known it.

• She has the right to reactions: of shock, fear, anger, guilt, anxiety, and depression; of abhorrence for a disease that has probably led to mutilation and will ultimately be lethal.
• She has a right to feel "contagious," "unwanted," "unclean." One woman asked: "Is cancer catching? Running through my mind after the operation was the idea that the staff was half afraid it was and weren't too pleased with having to get involved with personal nursing."
Another patient had a better experience: "In my case I was lucky. A nurse sat down and talked to me. She gave me a back rub. In short, she made me feel I was still part of the human race and not a newly discovered leper."
Many women wonder if they are still acceptable as sexual partners. A 62-year-old woman, usually very reserved, asked her physician six weeks before she died whether it would be all right for her to have sex with her husband. "I think Jack would like it," she said wistfully.
• The patient has a right to confidentiality. If it is her wish not to tell her husband or family or have the doctors or nurses do so, it is her right. Her wishes come first, although I admit it may be wise to help her see that those close to her should know. It goes without saying that she has the right to hear her diagnosis before anyone else is told.
• The patient has a right to be in such a state of shock that she doesn't hear—or grasp—what the doctor says the first time, the second, or the third. One woman commented that "two very nice doctors told me everything...but I've forgotten. Would you," she asked her physician "tell me again?" And when he had finished, she asked: "If I forget

again may I ask you to tell me once more?" She has, then, the right to have the information she wants repeated as often as she needs it to be.

• The patient has a right to show curiosity. In fact I believe that the patient should be encouraged to express curiosity and interest about her condition, the treatments that she will undergo, and the complications to her body and psyche that these treatments may produce now or later. She has the right if she wishes (and *only if she wishes*) to know the score—as many of the facts as she wants and can tolerate.

• The patient has a right to know the different medical procedures available and the doctor's preference for treatment. She may ask what he would do if she were his wife or daughter. She has a right to expect concern and good judgment. One patient commented: "I think there should be openness about what the doctor perceives to be the best possible treatment. But I think that a doctor should be aware of the intelligence and the emotional climate of the patient and not burden that patient with something she's not capable of handling. Thus, despite my doctor's conviction that I would not be able to tolerate the mutilation of a certain procedure because of my strong body image, I would have expected him to work with me until I could tolerate it if that were the very best thing for me."

• The patient has the right of autonomy over her own body. She can choose whether or not to have research or palliative treatment and if so, what method, where, and by whom. She has the right to refuse all treatment. She has the right to change her mind and be accepted again as a patient who will follow through as recommended. Many patients need time to mourn their plight before the new treatment starts. Expression should be encouraged, and no one should be rejected for having to think and feel things through. Some patients grieve quickly and others, as our good nurses know, express it simply and directly—usually by sadness and depression—the day before treatment.

• At all times, regardless of positive or questionable outcome, the patient should be able to accept the fact that the attending physician is the most important member of the treatment team. As a patient said, "Anybody who does not recognize this fact is only fooling or kidding herself." It is also essential that doctor and patient mutually approve of and respect one another. . .and if they do not, she has the right to change doctors.

• The patient has the right to be aware of, to receive, or to request psychological help. She should at the same time be sensitive to what type of mental health therapy is acceptable to the professionals caring for her and to her significant family members. One patient who sought help from a counselor during treatment commented: "The most help, apart from the doctors, was from my therapist because the struggle with one's self is more difficult than the struggle with one's body. He helped me toward a self-realization, to find my self-force, the courage."

• She should know that sometimes the very thing that hinders also helps—that these forces may overlap or change at some future time.

"My anxiety level was very hindering. Yet in a sense it was helpful. It forced me to get up and go to the treatment every day."

"The impersonality of the doctors at the clinic was distressing. I wished for more human contact, but sometimes it's easier to be brave and get through painful moments when you have to do it alone."

"I'm learning to live with uncertainty and seeing it as a kind of freedom."

"Telling you about my experience has been painful, but it is a way of helping other people that would not of course have been available to me or appropriate for me. It's also been a release, to get it out."

"I'm more aware of how I'd like to live."

• The patient has the right to know that she may take another important helping step: externalizing her cancer, giving a new form to the experience outside of the psyche. She should take or be given a method for expressing her feelings, such as drawing, painting, keeping a diary, verbal communication with a nurse, counselor, chaplain, physical therapist, or occupational therapist. Most of all, the patient has the right to be directed to these helpful people for a treatment regimen that may not directly relate to the actual medical procedure. Parallel assistance helps the patient to accept the medical treatment and to plan ahead.

One patient chose drawing and painting as a complement to mental health therapy. She said, "Pictures gave a new form to my feelings, to my loneliness. I got closer to my feelings, and suffering took a new form. I had deeper contact with myself."

• The patient has the right to express her wishes about the use of extraordinary measures for continuing her life and to expect those wishes to be respected. Although living wills are helpful, they are not enough. Each decision needs to be explored with the patient anew. Despite her earlier expectations, she might still want to cling to life.

The burden for everyone is greater when the disease is not checked or curable, during the long period when treatment is only a measure of prolonging life or easing pain. The patient can be a more effective partner in her own care if she understands what the doctor is going through—that his or her profession is closely bound to saving lives, not attuned to giving them up. The patient may be too self-pitying, too angry at the world and herself to understand, but I have found that the patient usually has more insight into the doctor's problem than he has himself. Generally the patient is competent if she wishes to exercise her rights as a preterminal or terminal patient.

In considering patient rights, expecially in the preterminal and terminal stages of her illness, it is important to remember that her illness is her private territory. No matter how much she loves and needs her friends and family, how close she feels to her professional helpers, everyone is an outsider to her experience. "You know, dear," one patient told her husband, "we are no longer partners. You see, I am dying and you are living and that is what separates us, closes us off, one from the other." It was in that spirit, when widespread infection made any further treatment merely palliative, that she declined treatment and "won the battle in her own way."

10

The Right to Choose
a Place to Die

William F. Finn

Does a patient have a right to choose where he will die? To answer this, we must distinguish between the wants and needs of the patient and his needs as these are defined by others, usually nurses or doctors. The wants of the patient may be unreasonable based on standards of feasibility for the family, the home, and the cost. The needs of the patient may be practical and achievable but also may exceed what is determined by the physician, the social service agency, and/or the government. The right to a choice of a place for dying, like the right to health care, exists (*Journal of Medicine and Philosophy*, 1979). But it may be compromised by the physical and emotional limitations of the dying person, the family's structure and financial means, support from agencies, and the type of available residence. The right to choose a place to die is moral rather than legal, extraordinary rather than ordinary, relative rather than absolute, and imperfect. It is based on the dying person, the family, the length and character of the dying process, the living quarters, and the financial independence of the family. It might be subjected to a cost/benefit analysis, but such appraisals are almost always unfavorable because so many of the benefits are imponderables. One shining hour can, in the eyes of the dying patient, outweigh thousands of dollars.

There are, it seems, four places where one can die: highway, hospital, hospice, and home.

Highway

This term is used to express death *away* from the hospital, the hospice, or the home. It encompasses the deaths on the farms and the hunting accidents of two decades ago, but a new dimension of high-velocity accident has been added, a consequence of airplanes and faster cars. Natural events such as hurricanes, tornadoes, and floods occur as in the past but other new dimensions of violence have been introduced into contemporary society. The murder of an intended victim or the death of the innocent bystander is recorded daily in our news media, as are deaths caused in mass disasters—of children in a school bus crushed at a train crossing, of passengers in an airplane crash, of workers trapped in a chemical factory explosion, or citizens on the scene when a building collapses. Our population is constantly exposed to immediate, unanticipated death or a condition of barely being alive, with rapid downgrade progression. Cardiac pulmonary resuscitation and other life-preserving modalities may be administered at the site of the accident or in the ambulance on the way to the hospital. Despite efforts bordering on the heroic, death occurs. Obviously, the right to choose where we will die does not exist for anyone dying on the "highway."

Hospital

Accident victims frequently are dead on arrival at the hospital emergency room. Some are barely alive even with support systems functioning at their highest efficiency. The dead and seriously injured may be victims of single or mass accidents. In the latter case, the resources—human and mechanical—of the emergency room may be severely taxed or even exceeded. Triage procedures and a priority list for scarce resources may have to be determined, including blood, respirators, and use of operating room facilities. The patient is usually unconscious and hence can exercise no choice. A conscious patient may be so weakened and impaired that he cannot make a rational choice. Analgesics may further impair judgment. The patient, while possessing vital signs, may have irreparable cortical brain death.

The patient may be taken from the emergency room to the operating room for stoppage of bleeding, repair of trauma, and setting of fractures. Analgesia and anesthesia preclude freedom of choice here. The unconscious patient may die without recovering consciousness. This might also happen in the recovery room or the surgical intensive care unit, but usually consciousness has returned. Repair of the traumatized body and mind begins. The patient will ultimately be moved to the general surgical medical ward where he can exercise more choice. Injuries may be so severe that there is small hope for a patient's survival. At times the length of the dying process permits rational choice. Where state laws do not recognize neurological death, despite irreversible damage to the cortex of the brain, only cessation of pulse and respiration are regarded as criteria of death.

Some accident patients are admitted directly to chronic medical and surgical areas with heart trouble, neurological and renal diseases, cancer, and other long-term, potentially fatal illnesses. For them, there may be many opportunities for decision-making, and patient, family, and physician can discuss and choose among options of treatment and place of care. Decisions can be reconsidered and reversed; patients can stay on a traditional program alternating between hospital and home, or they may (if terminal) wish to become part of a hospice/home program.

Hospice

Dissatisfaction with the medical and nursing care of dying patients or with the general medical and surgical areas of hospitals appears to have led to the institution of hospices as sites for caregiving between the home and the acute care hospital. Here the rules of the hospital are relaxed. Since hospice patients are dying, an attempt is made to treat them and the bereaved relatives as though they were at home. Visiting hours are extended; children, even infants, may visit. Favorite foods are brought in and fear of narcotic addiction is dispelled.

I favor hospices as an integral part of a hospital to permit access to the hospital resources. Government planning favors a hospice in a building near the hospital. While this gives the hospice a separate identity, it fails to provide backup support. If the physical structure of the hospice is separate from the hospital, it must be close enough to permit effective collaboration between hospital personnel and hospice personnel.

The hospice service usually starts as an outpatient department with visiting nurses and physicians who make house calls. Many patients can be cared for at home and almost all prefer to be there. North Shore University Hospital (Manhasset, New York) has a superb program where an oncology fellow, an oncology nurse, and a laboratory technician visit patients at home. Their vehicle is an ambulance with all life support systems and laboratory facilities, and their program supplements visits to hospital clinics and doctors' offices, as well as admissions to hospice or hospital.

Home

If they could, most patients would choose to die at home. Here they are with their family, with visiting relatives and friends. The patient is in familiar surroundings, in his own bed, looking forward to usual meals. There is television and radio without arbitrary time limits or lights out; a favorite easy chair or a window to watch the birds; and loved objects all around.

Certain characteristics are required of the patient, family, support system, home, and environment. The patient must have courage. He cannot complain about every ache and must accept setbacks. Pain must be controllable. The patient cannot be incontinent of urine or feces. There cannot be open, foul-smelling wounds, and the patient must be mentally alert.

The family has to love the patient and continue to demonstrate this love even after the patient in his terror becomes nasty, complaining, and uncooperative. There must be a mature, "unflappable" person, usually a wife, husband, or adult child. Patient care can be supplemented by housekeeper, nurses, aides, and so forth. With the loss of the extended family, we have lost what every family once had—the unmarried spinster aunt or the widowed grandmother who would take over.

Support systems are vital supplements to the patient and the family. They may be informal (relatives, neighbors, and friends who help the main provider). In addition, there are formal means of support such as Cancer Care, American Heart Association, and other organizations giving direct aid and referrals to other support sources.

Home care also requires certain minimum environmental standards: —a separate but unisolated bedroom, facilities for bathing the patient, laundry facilities. These can be found in a home, an apartment, or even a furnished room. But only love will make proper care possible.

Unfortunately, an essential ingredient for permitting a patient to exercise his right of choice is the financial ability to back his choice of a place to die. The poorer one is the more restricted one's choices; the richer, the wider one's choices. If one is very rich, one can sit on a Hawaiian hilltop like Charles Lindbergh and watch the Pacific Ocean and sky blur into nothingness as one's vital forces disappear.

Reference

Rights to Health Care. 1979. *The Journal of Medicine and Philosophy.* (June) 4.

Part III

Hospice Caregiving

11

Hospice Care: A Better Way of Caring for the Living

Pamela Gray-Toft and James G. Anderson

Hospice refers to an organized program that provides a continuum of home and inpatient care for the terminally ill patient and family. Palliative and supportive care are provided by an interdisciplinary team to alleviate the physical, emotional, spiritual, social, and economic stresses experienced by patient and family during the final stages of illness and during the bereavement period (National Hospice Organization 1978). Although originating in England, hospices have appeared in North America in a variety of forms. These include home-care programs, free-standing facilities, specialized units in acute care hospitals, and hospice teams that serve terminally ill patients throughout the hospital.

The purpose of this paper is to elucidate a number of contributions that the hospice concept has made to the health care scene, to look at some of the problems involved in implementing the concept, and to suggest a reformulation and wider application of the hospice approach based on a broader concept.

Contributions of the Hospice Concept

The hospice concept represents a significant medical innovation. It involves a program for the care of the terminally ill rather than just a specialized facility or unit for the dying. In its broadest sense, the hospice approach has significant implications for the organization and delivery of health care in the United States. In contrast to the almost exclusive emphasis on research, diagnosis, cure, and prolongation of life that characterizes the present health care system, hospice programs focus on the symptoms of disease and attempt to ensure that the remainder of the terminal patient's life is as comfortable and meaningful as possible. This is accomplished by providing palliative care to control the physical symptoms of the disease, by offering emotional and psychological support for the patient and family as they experience the psychosocial consequences of a terminal illness, and by ensuring continuity of care during the terminal stages of illness.

The first aspect that differentiates hospice care from more traditional health care is the shift in emphasis from cure to the medical management of physical symptoms, particularly pain, when cure is no longer feasible. The chronic pain experienced by many terminally ill patients is protopathic—constant, persistent, and intensifying over time. This unremitting pain requires treatment regimens that prevent pain rather than attempt to control it once it is present. Hospice programs attempt to prevent this pain, as well as secondary symptoms such as nausea, insomnia, incontinence, and constipation through the sophisticated use of analgesics and other measures such as radiotherapy, peripheral nerve or intrathecal block, neurosurgery, or physical measures (Mount et al., 1976).

A second innovative aspect of hospice care is the recognition of the psychosocial impact of terminal illness upon the patient and family. Emotional and psychological support for them is considered as important as symptom control. Hospice programs view the patient as part of a family system whose well-being affects and is affected by the care provided. Families are assisted in providing care for the patient at home as long as possible. During periods when this is not feasible and inpatient care is required, provisions are made to ensure the continuing involvement of the family. For example, the family is encouraged to assist the hospice staff in giving such care as feeding, turning, and bathing the patient. This may require unrestricted visitation policies and special arrangements for meals and overnight accommodations for family members. Support is offered for the family before and after the patient's death. This generally includes bereavement follow-up services such as attendance at the funeral, home visits, telephone calls, and letters to the family from the hospice staff member who had primarily cared for the patient.

A third innovation of hospice programs is the emphasis on continuous comprehensive care. Hospice care generally requires home care services supplemented by a variety of inpatient and social services. These services are coordinated by the formation of an interdisciplinary team that ideally includes physicians, nurses, social worker, chaplain, psychologist, dietitian, pharmacist, physiotherapist, and specially trained volunteers. This approach ensures that patients will not lose contact with the special symptom control measures, medication regimens, and support given by family and staff as they move in and out of a hospital or other inpatient facility during their terminal illness (Plant 1977).

Problems Involved in Implementing the Hospice Concept

The hospice movement has undoubtedly brought to public awareness the needs of the dying, as well as attempting to meet these needs. However, the contribution that the hospice concept can make to the health care system is currently limited by three factors. First, it is questionable whether the public and health care professionals are willing to support facilities and programs that rather narrowly focus on the provision of palliative and supportive care for the terminally ill. Second, the giving of emotional and psychological support to terminally ill patients and their families results in excessive stress for the hospice staff. Third, within the present health care system, it is difficult to offer the continuous comprehensive care that the hospice concept embodies.

These issues are illustrated with case material from a study of the hospice unit at Methodist Hospital of Indiana in Indianapolis. This hospice was created as an experimental unit under the auspices of the Department of Medical Research in July 1977. A year later it became a regular, eleven-bed unit of the hospital. It was relocated in a wing of an existing medical unit and a new nursing staff was recruited, oriented, and trained. The hospice staff consists of nine registered nurses, five licensed practical nurses, and four senior nursing assistants.

While this case material is from a specialized unit in an acute-care hospital, the problems identified are inherent in the hospice model. Furthermore, it appears that the future growth of the hospice movement will depend largely upon the development of hospital-based programs. Funds generally are not available for new facilities at a time when there appears to be an excess of general hospital beds (Cohen 1979, Holden 1979, Mount 1976). At the same time, the need for hospital-based programs is evident from health care statistics that indicate 61 percent of the deaths in the United States occur in hospitals and other institutions. Most of these deaths result from cardiovascular disease, malignant neoplasms, cerebrovascular disease, and respiratory disease (U.S. Department of Health, Education and Welfare 1965). The progression of these diseases involving a series of treatment modalities, successive periods of long-term hospitalization, gradual deterioration, and ultimate death makes these patients suitable candidates for hospice programs.

Lack of Support

Critics point out that the hospice movement's exclusive involvement with dying patients lacks support from physicians, as well as the public. This results from the limited hospice concept, which conflicts with a public policy designed to cure disease and prolong life through scientific investigation and the development of new technology (Rossman 1979: 191-93).

The health professions in general embody a system of values that emphasizes the preservation of life. Underlying this system is the belief that medical science should seek mastery over all medical problems. Death is considered an indication of failure. Studies have shown that physicians tend to cope with their anxiety by ordering unrealistic treatment and by avoiding dying patients and their families, leaving much of the responsibility for the patient's care to the nurse. They frequently neglect the patient's and family's requests for information about the medical condition and its prognosis (Price and Bergen 1977, Schulz and Aderman 1976, Siegler 1975, Sudnow 1967).

Support for the hospice movement is particularly a problem when hospice programs do not allow for active therapy alongside palliative and supportive care. This forces the physician, patient, and family, at some point, to make a decision that active therapy is no longer warranted. Having to tell patients that they are dying and no further active treatment is warranted is difficult for physicians.

The consequences of this dilemma were observed in the Methodist Hospital hospice study. Before patients are referred to the unit, they are supposed to be informed of their terminal status. Active therapy for symptom control is maintained for some patients. However, patients are not coded for resuscitation. As a result of these admission policies, physicians' use of the hospice is low. During the first year of operation of the hospice unit in Methodist Hospital, four oncologists admitted more than 70 percent of the 201 patients. In commenting on this problem, one hospice nurse observed: "It is very difficult to say to a patient, 'You are going to die.' The oncologists are better able to talk to terminally ill patients. Other doctors can't talk to them so they keep them on another floor to avoid the issue."

The unwillingness of physicians to refer patients to the hospice creates problems regarding the optimum use of beds. "Inappropriate" (that is, not terminally ill) patients may be admitted to the hospice when other hospital beds are full and there are vacant hospice beds. This results in considerable stress on the part of the hospice nurse regarding the presence of coded patients on the unit. They fear that if they resuscitated such a patient, it could lead to demands that they initiate heroic measures for terminally ill patients (Gray-Toft and Anderson 1980a).

Even when physicians refer patients to the hospice unit, they frequently fail to fully inform them of their terminal prognosis and of the nature of the hospice. This results in stress for the hospice nurse who has to effect the transfer from the other unit. One nurse commented that stress for her was the doctors' "copping out" of their responsibility to inform patients that their conditions were terminal. On occasion this leads to situations where the hospice staff is uncertain about what information the physician conveyed to the patient and family. This becomes more of a problem when family members turn to nurses to meet their needs for reassurance, information, and guidance.

Patients and their families are also frequently unwilling to relinquish their faith in the curative power of modern medicine and to agree to termination of active therapy prior to admission to a hospice program. An early study of cancer patients recognized this problem. The study recommended that specialized facilities for terminal cancer patients should not be developed. It stated that such units would produce severe emotional trauma for the patient and family (Institute of Medicine of Chicago 1950). It is noteworthy that British hospices do not care only for the terminally ill (St. Christopher's Hospice 1977).

Such trauma is poignantly illustrated by the reactions of one patient who had been informed of his terminal status by his physician and referred to the hospice unit at Methodist Hospital. The nurse who interviewed him prior to his admission to the unit gave the following account:

One day last week I went to interview a patient on our waiting list for hospice. The information we had about him stated that he was angry at his doctor for telling him he had cancer. I went into his room, a four-bed ward, and introduced myself. He said his doctor wanted him transferred. He never talked about hospice. I asked him what he knew about his condition. He said he had cancer of the lung and now it was in his kidney. I told him our patients were incurable. He became angry, said he was *not* incurable and did not want to be with *those* patients. He said that if he couldn't be cured at Methodist, he'd go to the clinic outside of Chicago that cured his brother-in-law. I told him that it was his choice and he could talk to his doctor again. Jan, the assistant head nurse, called one of the doctors following his case and she said that she would talk with him again because she wanted him on hospice. Later she (the doctor) came to the hospice and said that he *was* coming. It sounded like "by force." He was transferred in later that afternoon.

In order to avoid forcing the patient to give up all hope by terminating active therapy, some hospices in the United States provide more than palliative care. For example, Calvary Hospital in New York performs a clinical evaluation of each new patient. Active therapeutic measures are initiated in instances where curative possibilities have been overlooked, although no heroic measures are taken to prolong life. This procedure assures the patient that every effort has been made to cure him (Rossman 1979: 135).

Staff Stress

The giving of emotional and psychological support to terminally ill patients and their families is emotionally draining. Excessive stress leads to a high rate of burnout and turnover among hospice staff. This is particularly the case when the health professional has had little training in this area and when his/her patient load consists entirely of the dying. Balfour Mount, Director of the Palliative Care Service at the Royal Victoria Hospital, in a private correspondence has stated that all of the pioneering hospices experienced significant staff distress. He reported that job-related stress for health professionals working with dying patients in his own hospice unit had been dangerously high. It had resulted in severe depression, impaired social functioning, serious physical disorders, and marital breakdown.

The study of the hospice unit at Methodist Hospital (Gray-Toft and Anderson 1980b) indicated that nurses experienced stress as a result of their constant exposure to death and dying, as well as of a lack of professional support. They also felt inadequately prepared to offer emotional and psychological support to dying patients and their families. Additional stress for the hospice staff resulted from practices and policies designed to facilitate the provision of psychosocial care for the patient and family. These involved special physical facilities, staffing policies, visitation procedures, and scheduling of meals that differentiated the hospice from other, more traditional hospital units. Such practices and policies resulted in increased work load, a sense of isolation, and emotional demands on the hospice staff (Gray-Toft and Anderson 1980a).

Provision of Continuous Comprehensive Care

The third major problem involved in implementing the hospice concept revolves around the giving of continuing comprehensive care. Discontinuity is inherent in the hospice concept, as well as the result of restrictions imposed by the present health care system. In the United

States hospices are designed specifically for patients who have had a terminal diagnosis. Therefore, the initiation of hospice care frequently results in an abrupt discontinuation of therapeutic regimens and, in the case of hospitalized patients, physical transfer from one hospital unit to a specialized hospice facility.

Patients at Methodist Hospital are considered appropriate for hospice care when they are diagnosed as terminal with less than six months to live. At the discretion of the attending physician, patients may be offered the opportunity to transfer from their present hospital unit to the hospice, but transfer separates the patient and family from the nursing staff and sometimes from the physicians who have supplied care at the very time when continuity of support is paramount. This discontinuity in care results in a feeling of lack of support, and in some instances abandonment, in patients and families as can be seen in figure 11-1.

As part of the Methodist Hospital study, patients in five hospital units were asked to indicate on a Hospital Unit Atmosphere Scale (HUAS), developed by the authors, how much support they perceived from nurses, physicians, and other patients. Patients in all but the hospice unit perceived more support from physicians than from nurses or patients. In contrast, terminally ill patients in the hospice unit perceived the least support from physicians in dealing with their terminal illness (Gray-Toft and Anderson 1979).

Discontinuity also results from hospital reimbursement policies that require a patient to be discharged once his or her condition is no longer acute. This results in attempts to "con the system." Physicians may continue to certify a terminally ill patient's condition as acute after it has been successfully treated because the patient has nowhere to go. Physicians also report scattering their patients around the hospital to hide the fact that federal funds are being accepted for patient care to which the hospital is not technically entitled (Rossman 1979: 149).

The discharge of a patient to another institution because of suspension of insurance coverage frequently results in feelings of anger and guilt on the part of family members and a sense of loss by the nursing staff. This can be seen in the following account of a nurse's conversation with the wife of a terminally ill patient who had to be discharged from the Methodist Hospital to a VA hospital because his condition was no longer considered acute.

I said goodbye to Mary the night before Frank was to leave for the VA. She was very emotional and confronted me with several questions which I couldn't answer. "Why does he have to go to a nursing home? I wouldn't send a dog to a nursing home. He's suffered for 10 years. Why can't he stay where he's loved and cared for?"

Shortly after the transfer hospice nurses stated that they felt it was unfair to let a patient die in another institution when they had invested so much in the patient and family. They also felt that their work was left "unfinished."

Providing continuous medical and psychosocial care once the patient has left the hospital also presents problems. The present health care system is poorly designed for such care. A number of separate agencies must be involved in the comprehensive care that hospice programs attempt to supply. This results in problems of coordination and continuity.

The offering of comprehensive care is made even more difficult by current third-party reimbursement policies. A recent survey of insurance companies indicated that only 17 percent pay hospice benefits. Generally the only services that are reimbursable are medical nursing health services involving the "laying on of hands." Benefits for counseling, bereavement services, and social work are almost nonexistent (Cohen 1979: 101-23; Rossman 1979: 214-17).

Toward a Broader Application of the Hospice Concept

The previous sections have discussed some of the innovative aspects of hospice care and some of the problems involved in implementing the concept. The remainder of this paper outlines a way in which the hospice concept could be broadened to have much wider application and a greater impact upon the health care system. A survey of the literature and a case study of the Methodist Hospital hospice suggest that some of the problems involved in fulfilling the hospice concept in the United States are the result of having too narrow a view of hospice, namely, of limiting hospice care to the dying patient. It would seem that several of the disadvantages of hospice as it now stands could be minimized and the advantages of hospice care maximized by extending the concept to all patients faced with life-threatening and terminal illness.

One way that this could be accomplished is through the development of a hospital-based continuing health care center. Continuing health care is not viewed just as posthospital care but as encompassing all those services—inpatient, outpatient, day and home care—required at any point in the continuum of health and medical care (McNamara 1978). The creation of such a center within the general hospital would be designed to balance the current emphasis on life-saving services oriented toward short-term acute care. It would include a broad range of services designed to help people cope with the stress associated with life-threatening and terminal illnesses.

Components of a Continuing Health Care Program

The essential components of a continuing health care program are as follows:

1. Physically, it is part of a general hospital.
2. It is committed to research, diagnosis, and cure. Where cure is not possible, symptom control is emphasized.
3. It serves patients and families faced with life-threatening and terminal illness requiring multiple treatment modalities and repeated hospitalization that often result in protracted dying. Patients with the following diseases would be appropriate for such a program: renal failure, congestive heart failure, cancer, emphysema, cystic fibrosis.
4. The program emphasizes the treatment of patients within their family system.
5. It assumes responsibility for the provision of continuous care for patients from the time of diagnosis through treatment, with bereavement follow-up for family members. To facilitate continuous care and to encourage family care of the patient, the program incorporates a home-care service, day care facilities, and outpatient facilities in addition to inpatient and extended care facilities. When cure is no longer feasible, patients and families are not separated or physically relocated but continue to be given palliative and supportive care by the same health professional team.
6. It supplies comprehensive care whereby all resources are used to

implement a holistic approach to health care. The patient is treated by a team of professionals, including physicians, nurses, psychologist, social worker, chaplain, dietitian, pharmacist, and physiotherapist. Community resources, including specially trained volunteers and self-help programs, are used to assist in care. A comprehensive patient and family education program is offered. The entire program recognizes the psychosocial effects of disease and the effects of psychological processes upon disease and treatment. It gives psychological care at the point when chronic or terminal disease is first a reality rather than a last resort at the end phase of life when there is no hope of cure.

7. Staff education programs are offered in recognition of the need to educate health professionals in the wholistic approach to the treatment of life-threatening and terminal illnesses.

8. Staff support programs are an integral part of the program in order to alleviate the stress that results in burnout and turnover among health professionals who continuously care for chronic and terminal patients.

Advantages of a Continuous Health Care Model

The proposed continuing health care model is broader and has a number of significant advantages over the hospice model. First, research, diagnosis, cure, and prolongation of life are important components of the model. In providing care for patients, all available treatment modalities will be used, as well as any new therapeutic or curative advances.

Second, it recognizes and attends to the psychological and emotional effects of disease at the point when chronic disease or terminal disease is first a reality. The patient is confronted with his or her mortality and supported through the process of adjusting to this and to the limitations imposed by the disease. Psychosocial care is seen as an important part of medical care. At the outset the physician recognizes and assists the patient to understand that all attempts to cure or maintain the patient will be made but that, at the same time, medical science has its limitations.

The model clearly recognizes that the way patients respond psychologically to life-threatening or terminal illness not only influences the course of the disease and the effectiveness of treatment but also presents major problems for the hospital staff (Cohen and Lazarus 1979). In addition, it recognizes the patient's and family's need for support in coping with the psychosocial consequences of a life-threatening illness at all stages. While hospice programs attempt to give care and support at the terminal stage, the present health care system supplies little in the way of support for individuals and their families at the onset of a life-threatening illness.

A number of advantages stem from this broader continuing health care model. In contrast to a hospice one would expect greater acceptance and therefore greater use by the public and health care professionals. This facility is not a "death house," although some patients are dying. The physician and patient are not forced at a single point in time to make a decision that requires the physical transfer of the patient to a terminal unit when cure is no longer deemed possible.

The wholistic approach to health incorporated in this model is challenging. It offers an opportunity for health professionals to recapture the idealism that initially attracted many of those who later became disenchanted with the fragmented and limited concept of care that characterizes the current health care system.

Furthermore, the recognition and earlier attention to the psychosocial needs of the patient and family should result in a significant reduction in the stress experienced by the nursing and medical staff compared to that occurring when support is provided only at the terminal stage. This would particularly be the case if physicians and nurses were educated to believe that prolongation of life regardless of quality is not preferable and that the death of a patient is not failure when all possible curative therapies have been exhausted. Stress reduction would also result from the inclusion of patients at all stages of illness, not merely the terminal phase.

Third, the continuing health care model assumes responsibility for the provision of continuous comprehensive care at all stages of a life-threatening or terminal illness. Whereas the hospice model emphasizes continuous comprehensive care, in actual fact, it is unable to provide such care. As discussed earlier, this is partly the result of the exclusive concern with dying patients that gives rise to sharp discontinuities in the giving of care. In contrast, the continuing health care model ensures greater continuity of care by supplying inpatient, extended, outpatient, day, and home care.

The location of the continuing health care center within the hospital recognizes the fact that the general hospital is the one institution capable of assuming responsibility for the offering of the comprehensive health services that the hospice concept embodies. Such a central role for the hospital has been advocated for more than a decade (National Commission on Community Health Services 1967, 37th American Assembly 1970, Somers 1971) and was implicit in legislation that led to the Regional Medical Program in 1965 (President's Commission on Heart Disease, Cancer and Stroke 1964).

Another major advantage of the proposed continuing health care model results from its potential effect on the use of acute-care beds. The offer of alternative types of care for large numbers of chronically and terminally ill patients could result in a reduction in acute-care beds and their conversion to other uses such as long-term care. In addition, continuing care services would alleviate some of the need for the construction of additional acute-care hospital beds (Osterweis and Champagne 1979).

Implementation of a Continuous Health Care Model

The creation of a hospital-based continuing health care center and the implementation of these recommendations would require a number of changes in the present health care system. First, it would require the establishment of a structured relationship between primary care and hospital care for reasons of both economy and quality. This dichotomy presently underlies the fragmentation that characterizes not only the United States health care system but also most European systems (Somers 1970).

Under this proposal the general hospital through the continuing health care center would assume responsibility for providing the full range of comprehensive health services required by this program. Ideally this would be accomplished by the creation of a center within the hospital consisting of the components outlined above. In communities where this is not feasible the hospital would be the operational center of an integrated network of community health services.

A second important factor in implementing this program involves changes in current third-party reimbursement policies. At present no comprehensive health insurance plan exists that specifically covers hospice-type services. Reimbursement for inpatient or home care services at present does not cover most aspects of psychosocial care such as bereavement care, counseling, or social services. Furthermore these policies do not recognize the hospice concept of providing care for the family as a unit. Services for family members are not reimbursable unless each individual is covered by Medicare, Medicaid, or some other insurance program (Rossman 1979: 214-17). As a result, many of the services that constitute the continuing health care program that is proposed would have to be paid for in most part by the patient and his family.

At present there are several experiments in hospice reimbursement. Blue Cross organizations in Genesee Valley, New York; and Washington, D.C., are examining modified reimbursement policies for a home care program and for an inpatient hospice program, respectively (Osterweis and Champagne 1979). Also, the Health Care Finance Administration has initiated several demonstration projects with organizations providing hospice services (USDHEW, 1978). For certain hospice services that are not adequately covered under the present policies, these projects grant waivers of Medicare coverage and reimbursement requirements and exclusions.

Both the federal government and commercial carriers need to carefully examine the feasibility of modifying reimbursement policies to include the full range of continuing health care services proposed here. Evidence is beginning to accrue that a hospice-type program that directly involves the patient and family in giving their own care while at the same time provides comprehensive continuing care can effectively reduce health care costs (Rossman 1979: 210-14). Part of the savings results from the substitution of home care and other services for acute care; part results from family counseling and bereavement care, which has been shown to be effective in reducing the psychosocial impact of a terminal illness on surviving family members (Parkes 1972).

Third, the proposed continuing health care model requires special selection and education of the health professionals and volunteers who staff such centers. There is increasing recognition of the effects of stress on health care providers (Cartwright 1979, Gray-Toft and Anderson 1980a, b). Special selection, an intensive period of specialized training prior to service, continuous inservice education, and a staff support program are essential if staff burnout, job dissatisfaction, and turnover are to be minimized. At Methodist Hospital a support program for hospice nurses was effective in reducing stress, increasing job satisfaction, and preventing burnout (Gray-Toft 1980a). It is especially important in continuing health care centers to decrease staff turnover in order to provide true continuity of care for patients with multiple admissions.

This paper has presented a model that broadens the hospice concept to include patients confronted with life-threatening and terminal disease at the point of initial diagnosis. Ideally the concept should be extended further, for it is nothing more than good medical care. We have proposed that hospice care be considered as a better way of caring for the living. In so doing, we would eliminate many of the disadvantages of hospice as it now stands and bring to the American health scene a sorely needed integration of a more humane way of caring for the ill.

References

American Assembly. 1970. *The Health of Americans.* Report of the 37th American Assembly. New York: Arden House.

Cartwright, L. K. 1979. "Sources and Effects of Stress in Health Careers." In G. C. Stone, F. Cohen and N. E. Alder eds., *Health Psychology.* San Francisco: Jossey-Bass, pp. 419-46.

Cohen, F. and R. S. Lazarus. 1979. "Coping with the Stresses of Illness." In G. C. Stone, F. Cohen and N. E. Alder eds., *Health Psychology.* San Francisco: Jossey-Bass, pp. 217-54.

Cohen, K. P. 1979. *Hospice: Prescription for Terminal Care.* Germantown, Md.: Aspen Systems Corporation.

Gray-Toft, P. A. 1980a. "Effectiveness of a Counseling Support Program for Hospice Nurses." *Journal of Counseling Psychology.* 27:346-54.

Gray-Toft, P. A. 1980b. "Coping with the Stress of Nursing Terminal Patients in a Hospice: Design, Implementation and Evaluation of a Staff Support Program." Paper prepared for the National Symposium on "The Role of the Community Hospital in Dealing with Life-threatening Disease and Bereavement," Bethlehem, Pa.: Foundation of Thanatology (January 10-12).

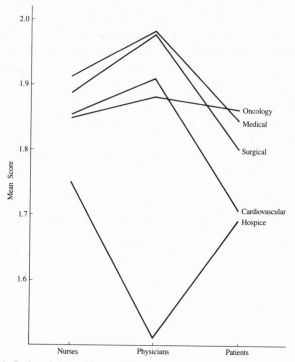

Figure 11-1. Patients' Perceptions of Support Received from Physicians, Nurses, and Other Patients

Gray-Toft, P. A. and J. G. Anderson. 1979. "A Study of Hospital Staff Stress: Sources of Stress and the Design and Evaluation of a Staff Support Program." Paper prepared for the National Seminar on Community Cancer Care, Indianapolis, Indiana (June 13).

Gray-Toft, P.A. and J.G. Anderson. 1980a. "Stress among Hospital Nursing Staff: Its Causes and Effects." *Social Science and Medicine* 15A:639-47.

Gray-Toft, P.A. and J.G. Anderson. 1980b. "Sources of Stress in Nursing Terminal Patients in a Hospice." Paper prepared for the National Symposium on "The Role of the Community Hospital in Dealing with Life-threatening Disease and Bereavement," Bethlehem, Pa.: Foundation of Thanatology (January 10-12).

Holden, C. 1976. "Hospices: For the Dying, Relief from Pain and Fear. *Science*. 193:389-91.

Institute of Medicine of Chicago. 1950. *Terminal Care for Cancer Patients*. Chicago: Central Service for the Chronically Ill.

McNamara, E. M. 1978. "Continuing Health Care: Attention Turns to Day Care and Hospice Services." *Hospitals J.A.H.A.* 52:79-83.

Mount, B. M., I. Ajemian, and J. F. Scott. 1976. "Use of the Brompton Mixture in Treating the Chronic Pain of Malignant Disease." *Canadian Medical Association Journal*. 115:122-24.

Mount, B. M. 1976. "The Problem of Caring for the Dying in a General Hospital: The Palliative Care Unit as a Possible Solution." *Canadian Medical Association Journal* 115:119-21.

National Hospice Organization. 1978. *Hospice Standards.* McLean, Va.: National Hospice Organization Standard and Accreditation Committee.

National Commission on Community Health Services. 1967. *Health is a Community Affair.* Cambridge, Mass.: Harvard University Press.

Osterweis, M. and D. S. Champagne. 1979. "The U.S. Hospice Movement: Issues in Development." *American Journal of Public Health.* 69:492-96.

President's Commission on Heart Disease, Cancer, and Stroke. 1964. *Report to the President* (December).

Parkes, C. M. 1972. *Bereavement.* New York: International Universities Press.

Plant, J. 1977. "Finding a Home for Hospice Care in the United States." *Hospitals J.A.H.A.* 51:53-62.

Price, T. R. and B. J. Bergen. 1977. "The Relationship to Death as a Source of Stress for Nurses on a Coronary Care Unit." *Omega* 8:229-38.

Rossman, P. 1979. *Hospice: Creating New Models of Care for the Terminally Ill.* New York: Fawcett Columbine Books.

St. Christopher's Hospice. 1977. *Annual Report, 1976-1977.* Sydenham, London.

Schulz, R. and D. Aderman. 1976. "How the Medical Staff Copes with Dying Patients: A Critical Review." *Omega* 7:11-21.

Siegler, M. 1975. "Pascal's Wager and the Hanging of Crepe." *New England Journal of Medicine* 293:853-57.

Somers, A. R. 1970. "Study of Care in Sweden and England Shows: The Hospital Is the Core of the System." *Modern Hospital* 115:87-91.

Somers, A. R. 1971. *Health Care in Transition: Directions for the Future.* Chicago: Hospital Research and Educational Trust.

Sudnow, D. 1967. *Passing On: The Social Organization of Dying.* Englewood Cliffs, N. J.: Prentice Hall.

U.S. Department of Health, Education, and Welfare. 1965. Public Health Service, National Center for Health Statistics. Hospitalization in the Last Year of Life—1961, series 22, No. 1. Washington, D.C.: U.S. Government Printing Office.

U.S. Department of Health, Education, and Welfare. 1978. Medicare and Medicaid Hospice Projects. *Federal Register* (October 27) 43, 50:376-78.

12

Relating to the Dying:
A Philosophy
of Continuing Care

Dean B. Pratt and Roberta Filicky-Peneski

Over the last several decades, the science of medicine has advanced rapidly while developments in the art of medicine have often lagged. The focus of scientific medicine has often been on the disease rather than the patient, and we medical professionals have found ourselves doing things to and for our patients rather than with them. Although caring may not have disappeared totally from the scientific aspect of medicine, it has often been disguised as doing. Doing to and for our patients in the cure-oriented society in which we live has often led us to miss that point in the course of a patient's disease beyond which further curative efforts seem inappropriate and even meddlesome.

Because of our failures in the art of medicine, many of us feel inadequate in dealing with patients as whole beings, particularly in situations of impending death. We often find it difficult to cope with the implications of death and to maintain a caring relationship with the dying patient.

We now find ourselves in search of innovative ideas for continuing care for the dying. If we want to talk about caring, there are three aspects of the philosophy of continuing care that we believe are mandatory no matter how the administrative structure is designed or what it is called. The first is a commitment to continued personal growth on the part of the caregivers; the second is structural flexibility; and the third is caring.

I (D.B.P.) have spent a considerable amount of time over the last years thinking about death and dying, talking about it, and learning to put my philosophy into practice. I have found that my philosophy has permeated my relationships with other patients and with my friends and acquaintances. Indeed, it has permeated all that I am and do. I am a different person today than I was three years ago, but I am not yet who or what I want to be. When I shall have arrived, the goals will have changed and I will need to continue the search, maintaining my commitment to continued personal growth.

The second aspect of continuing care is flexibility. Since the human organism is flexible, the social structures into which human beings are placed must be flexible. Laws and protocols are a necessary part of our social structures, designed to keep order. Too often we follow them to the letter, at great disregard for the patient. We must learn to relate to the *spirit* of those laws and protocols.

Perhaps the most important aspect of continuing care is that it must be truly *caring*. Caring is many things: it is a sense of humor, recognizing our own feelings and dealing with them appropriately, an attitude of self-confidence and self-worth, trusting in our own intuition. Caring is a touch, it is love, it is time, it is understanding. It has been said that to be a good teacher (physician? nurse?) one must first like one's self. Caring is truly liking yourself! Caring is conveyed through communication, honest, open, two-way, verbal, and nonverbal communication. If there is caring that is not communicated, it does not exist.

Commitments to continued personal growth, flexible social structures, and true caring are some of the obvious yet often overlooked "innovative" aspects of continuing care that we are in search of. We are obliged to teach these aspects along with the technical aspects of the protocols of continuing care. We believe the cornerstone of caring is communication; we can teach that essential through staff development programs. We must acknowledge that we all are students—whether physician, nurse, volunteer, patient, custodian, or secretary—as we all are also teachers. We must design programs for the development of the entire staff that teach three basic things: first, what is essential—that is, personal growth; second, communication—those verbal and nonverbal cues and their implications; and finally we must teach what death is teaching our patients—the value of time, focusing, and letting go.

13

Preserving Sexuality, Privacy and Personhood, Among the Chronically Ill and Dying

Mary Romano

It is not easy to combine respect for sexuality with care for those with preterminal or terminal illnesses or chronic diseases. Even the language used to talk about people who are ill desexualizes them. Men and women who use our various professional services are "patients," and that word (coming from a root meaning "to suffer") offers no differentiation among male and female patients and young patients.

We speak of people who are ill by diagnosis: the cardiac, the myocardial infarction, the quadriplegic. This "patientness" precludes sexuality, which itself is a celebration of life. Neoplastic and other chronic diseases in a sense imply a *termination* of life, producing a conflict between dying, on one side, and preserving sexuality and needs for privacy and intimacy among patients on the other.

Other problems involve the interface among health care institutions, patients, and their families. The patient and family come to the health care provider for cure, diagnosis, and relief, and for wellness. They endow caregivers with enormous power, and we, within the institution, to some degree accept that power. However, when we can no longer provide the diagnosis or the curative process, we find a loss of fantasy—a loss of dream. That loss engenders frustration, anger, and guilt.

Inherent in the nature of institutions is the depersonalization of self. Becoming a patient is becoming less of a breadwinner, homemaker, father or mother, spouse, son, or daughter. Yet in order for an individual to maintain sexuality, his or her roles must be maintained.

One way to maintain roles is to bring family into the health caregiving setting, but such a situation sets up conflicts among patient, family, and staff. Who is loyal to whom? Who is supposed to nurture, to discipline? These areas of conflict underlie much of the stress of caring for chronically or terminally ill patients.

Being in an institution means giving up privacy. Doors do not lock and curtains are difficult to close and open. A patient in a sense cedes the right to make space for himself, and he also opens new areas of personal intimacy not ordinarily discussed in social interactions. With the diagnosis of chronic or terminal illness, the patient's body is open to the scrutiny of many concerned people. As patients, we accept that concern and scrutiny in the spirit in which it is given. Yet, to be poked and prodded, questioned and requestioned, and moved about are invasions we consider peculiar in normal social exchange.

If we go to the supermarket and stand in someone's way, it would be unusual for that person to literally lift us up and turn us 90° to the right. In hospitals, people on stretchers and in wheelchairs are moved from place to place in the alteration of control that comes with patienthood. It is a paradox: strangers become intimate with the body *without* intimacy, and there are no magic solutions to eliminate the problem.

At what point do health care providers take over for family, and at what point does family take over for the care providers? When do patients have a voice in what goes on; when are they outvoted and by whom? These are the issues in preserving sexuality and needs for the privacy and intimacy of the chronically ill or dying. So often the ultimate fear is abandonment. (What will happen if my wife leaves me?) Fears are manifested in many ways, but one cannot get angry at a staff member for fear of retaliation through the withholding of pain medication, for example.

At the same time, caregivers themselves need "to abandon." Even Mother Theresa goes on retreat, an acknowledgment of the need for space for the staff *and* family members. By its very nature, 24-hour health care gives little opportunity for anybody's space.

Who sets limits on inappropriate behavior within the hospital or defines it—staff, the families, or the recipients of care? It is *not* appropriate, for example, for those in general medical and surgical settings to act out conflicts between their own levels of fatigue and their concerns for others. In work with chronically ill or terminally ill people, the conflict becomes even more difficult because patients' vulnerabilities compound the deliverers'.

How do we say to someone who is chronically ill or dying, "Listen, I'm bushed! I was up until 3 A.M. working on my income tax and I don't know what to do." To admit fatigue to ourselves and to the chronically ill and dying becomes extremely difficult.

As we move into hospice care and other models for the chronically ill and dying, we face a tremendous potential conflict of preserving the personhood of our ill men and women, their families, and ourselves.

14

Humor and Laughter– Their Role in Improving the Quality of Life and of Care

Alfons Deeken

For many or at least for some patients, a sense of humor can contribute greatly to making the final stage of life more meaningful, serene, and human. Of course, in a pluralistic society, dying patients reflect many values and have different needs. We in the caregiving professions are in constant danger of trying to generalize and categorize, fitting every patient into the same mold, and pretending that we know best what every patient needs. A pluralistic approach refrains from forcing a generalized treatment upon the dying patient and attempts to be open to the individual psychological needs of each patient, encouraging him to live his final period of life in a personal manner and to die his own personal death in accordance with his own ideas and ideals. Not every patient has to go through Kübler-Ross' five stages of dying, and not every patient may find help and consolation in the prospect of immortality. But if a certain medicine is not therapeutic for all patients, there should be no reason to withhold it from those whose psychosomatic health may be improved by it.

It is within this framework of an individualized, pluralistic approach to the dying that humor and laughter may be a much-neglected yet important help to improve quality of life. Our general culture tends to overemphasize the serious and grossly neglect humor and laughter. There is no lack of superficial merrymaking, but that is frequently an attempt to escape from the boredom of the serious business of life. The shallowness of this posture becomes ever more evident as man's life approaches its end.

Humor is an expression and reflection of the infinite richness of joyful human life itself; it is a creative force of so many varieties that like life itself it eludes definition. Etymologically, the English word *humor* comes from the Latin "humor" (plural: humores). Medieval doctors referred to the "fluids" in the human body as "humores" that give life to man. For them, humores were not accidental but vital essences, the "juice and sap of life" whose flow gives vitality to a person and which as a creative force is constantly recharging human life.

The poet W. H. Auden claims that successful living must pay respect to three worlds: work, worship, and carnival. One rarely reads about the importance of humor and laughter for the patient facing death, and yet, if humor and laughter are essential elements of life, they should never be ignored or forgotten. The persons most influential in creating the proper habitat for the dying are doctors and nurses. If we measure them according to Auden's triple standard of a genuinely human life there is no doubt that most doctors and caregivers of the dying are hardworking. As to worship, doctors and nurses are probably on the whole as religious as any other group. However, according to one doctor commenting on the words of Auden, physicians feel most uncomfortable in the world of carnival. "We blame our uneasiness on many things— dealing with death, fatigue, malpractice threats. Thus, we can easily excuse ourselves for leaving no time for laughter" (*Journal of The American Medical Association*, Dec. 21, 1979, p. 2765). Humor and laughter are essential ingredients of living; they become even more important in times of sickness as a healing balm, a medicine for the whole person.

Norman Cousins' *Anatomy of an Illness* advocates laughter as an important medical tool, as a powerful weapon in the war against disease. Cousins claims that through administering massive doses of laughter to himself he produced positive emotions and changes in his body chemistry that significantly contributed to his physical recovery. Ten minutes of genuine belly laughter had an anesthetic effect and gave him more than two hours of pain-free sleep. This laughter theory is based on scientific data showing that laughter enhances respiration and helps oxidize the blood.

Humor and laughter could become an important answer or partial solution to the following problems:

1. Death-fear—fear-reducing humor based on belief in immortality.

Fear of death is a common phenomenon among people approaching death. To a certain degree it is a healthy defense mechanism. However, too many people are burdened with excessive depressing fears. For them, a healthy dose of humor may be helpful as a fear-releasing therapy that will reduce their anxieties to a normal level.

Thomas More is one of the finest examples of a person who could joke minutes before his execution. In a spirit of teasing banter he told the man waiting with the ax that his neck was rather short and that he should hit carefully since his honor as executioner was at stake. Then he moved his beard from the execution block with the joking remark that his beard had not offended his King, Henry VIII, and therefore should not be cut off.

The jesting behavior of Thomas More indicates that he had transcended his fear of death and had acquired a serene sense of inner freedom and composure. His firm belief in life after death allowed him to express humorous thoughts even in the face of death, for he was able to view life and death from the perspective of eternity.

2. Stress and tension—humor and laughter as release of tension.

Going through life-threatening illnesses, patients usually suffer from great stress and multiple tensions. To a certain degree, these emotions seem to be healthy coping mechanisms. However, constant stress and tension over an extended period of time can have a debilitating effect on the already weakened patient. Humor, laughter, and joking can fulfill a tension-relieving function.

According to Immanuel Kant, sudden relief from tension is the key to all humor. He defines humor as "an affection arising from a strained expectation being suddenly reduced to nothing."

3. Aggression, anger, and hostility—humor and laughter as a cathartic reduction in the intensity of the aggressive feelings.

Kübler-Ross describes anger as the second in the five-stage process of dying. Although I do not agree with the view that all patients go through a stage of anger, nevertheless, feelings of aggression, anger, and hostility are quite frequent among people with a life-threatening disease. Encouraging the patient to develop a sense of humor and laughter could be for some a significant help in reducing the feelings of hostility.

4. Tendency to become passive—humor and laughter as stimulus to activity and human growth.

There is a natural tendency for the patient approaching death to become passive and to let the process of dying just happen. Our task in caregiving is to encourage the patient to search for a proper balance between the unavoidable passive posture and a personal adherence to an active control over the last period of life. Humor and laughter can stimulate the active and creative forces of man. It is significant that Freud considered humor as the hallmark of maturity.

5. Isolation and loneliness of the dying patient—community-forming power of humor and laughter.

Growing isolation and loneliness are for many patients the most painful experiences of the dying process. Not only do relatives generally visit less frequently as the patient approaches his final hours, but also several surveys indicate that even doctors and nurses decrease the number of visits when there is no hope of recovery. Thus, many patients are deprived of human companionship precisely at the time when they need it most.

The loneliness of the dying patient is a complex and multifaceted problem. Many patients may not even care about humor at this stage of life. However, numerous patients at this stage do appreciate humor and laughter as a means of human communication and are greatly helped by it. Laughing together creates a feeling of solidarity and community. It may not be a remedy for all patients, but for some dying persons, humor and laughter may be an important way of counteracting and overcoming the growing isolation and loneliness.

6. "Burned-out" cases among doctors and nurses dealing with dying patients—humor and laughter as preventive medicine and therapy for the caregivers.

Constant work with the dying may become a heavy emotional

strain; the number of "burned-out" cases in the caregiving professions is relatively high. Evidently the people giving constant help to the dying need help themselves. Developing a sense of humor and laughter may help them lessen the tension and create a more relaxed atmosphere.

Part IV

Helping the Dying:
Caregiver Approaches

15

A Nursing Perspective on Patient Care

Florence S. Wald

Over the past two decades, members of the nursing profession have taken on two significant new roles in addition to those of doctor's helpers in the hospital. In their traditional roles, they served as orchestrators of patient care settings and providers of home care as visiting nurses. The new nursing roles are those of the clinical nurse specialist and the family practitioner. Members of the interdisciplinary health care team can misjudge a particular nurse's potential contribution to the team. Obviously, each nurse does not have every talent in equal proportion. Assessing her strengths and weaknesses with a task to be done is essential in forming the interdisciplinary team. But nursing is a profession in transition.

The nurse's special contribution to any interdisciplinary effort for patients is twofold. The nurse does for patients what they cannot do for themselves, always with the objective to help them do it for themselves and become independent. Virginia Henderson (1966) has defined the nurse as the link between the doctor and the patient, often reconciling the perspective of the patient and the perspective of the doctor so that the problems and the treatments are agreed upon by all. In the care of patients with terminal illness, the nurse assists the patient in the crucial but difficult task of deciding between two antithetical approaches. On the one hand, there is curative treatment, and on the other there is palliative. Patients need an open system that provides both care and cure, so that the patient is assured a choice throughout the course of illness. The necessity of continuity in coordination requires an organizational structure that links institutions and caregivers in them. The patient's life-style must be respected and maintained. Throughout the illness and after the patient's death, help for the family is as important as care for the patient.

Palliative treatment has grown by leaps and bounds since Cicely Saunders' work began in 1963. Symptom control is crucial. The physician prescribing for the pain and trauma of surgery views things differently from the one who prescribes to deal with chronic pain or malignant tissue. The fears of addiction and the fantasy about what morphine, cocaine, and heroin can do are deeply embedded in caregivers and patients, and there has been resistance to change.

As new information about palliative treatment has been unfolding to reveal the true mechanism and management of pain, the relationship of psyche and soma, the understanding of ways to support the bereaved, spiritual care, and environment have gained recognition as therapeutic tools. And there is recognition that there must be care for the caregivers too.

While we as comforters have been learning palliative skills, intensive treatment for cancer has also changed. Early diagnosis has become more reliable. The relative values of surgery, radiation, and chemotherapy have been reassessed, and there is increasing candor among health professionals about what we know and what we do not. Physicians are now expected to share what they know with patients and family and to share decisions with them as well. We have and can give a more honest and accurate appraisal of what medicine can and cannot do with respect to both care and cure.

Vital statistics advise us that if the cancer can be diagnosed before it metastasizes, the chance of survival improves. But the doubling time of the cancer cell determines how long it takes to form a palpable lump of cancer cells. In the case of the fastest growing cancer of the breast, it may take 1,000 days, nearly three years, to reach that stage. Thus, the likelihood of cancer cells finding their way into lymph channels in those three years is high. Prognosis becomes uncertain even when diagnosis is early and treatment is immediate. Correct diagnosis and choice of treatment are imprecise in curative or palliative treatment. The transport of cells is not just through the lymph system, as previously thought. Once cancer cells get into the blood stream, spread of the disease is far more difficult to control. The multiple approaches now available for diagnosing and monitoring the cancer, including mammograms and CAT scans, when used in addition to traditional physical examinations and x-rays, increase the chances of knowing how far the cancer may have spread. Taking diagnosis step by step, the lumpectomy, first in the case of breast cancer, can also lead to a more reasonable pace in diagnosis and allow both physician and patient to consider alternatives together.

There have been changes in attitudes toward the complex problem of what and how to tell a patient. Every patient needs an explanation of his illness that will be understandable and convincing to him if he is expected to cooperate in treatment or be relieved of the burden of unknown fears. We are beginning to see the differences between people: how much they talk, how verbal they are, how reliable their hearing is, how much they speak the same language, and how much information they need at a particular time to bring their coping behavior to the optimum level.

Negotiating between these two systems—the care system and the cure system—is one of the most complex tasks regardless of what form any organization takes. It needs skill, clarity, maturity, honesty, and sensitivity. Negotiations between clinician and clinician, service and service, and institution and institution begin with being as effective in practice as possible and then being clear about the illness and what each treatment can and cannot do. This means maintaining and improving our skills, critiquing ourselves, and accepting criticism from others in judging how effective a treatment approach is.

Giving support to patient, family, and other caregivers who are engaged in care and accepting support is often difficult. Nurses have yet to solve the problem of how to give effective support to doctors. Most doctors have yet to learn that they need support and that it is all right to accept it. Team work requires mutual trust, respect, and commitment. Barriers in the medical world and the ambivalence of nurses who are changing their roles from doctors' helpers to professionals responsible and accountable for their acts make team work tricky.

Considerable stress and strain have been found between groups of caregivers when a patient is shifted from a curative to palliative treatment. It is manifest in blame, guilt, and mistrust before and during the referral process. After the referral, those palliative caregivers who are taking over the caregiving from the curative caregivers feel abandoned by and estranged from them. Attempts to keep the relationship open often generate resistance in the caregivers who have put heart, elbow grease, and endless hours into the care they gave, only to end in "failure." Doctors have an additional problem: They do not think it is good etiquette to continue to see a patient once another physician takes over that care.

Those giving curative treatment and those giving palliative treatment face the same unanswerable question: How long will this go on? Oliver Cope, while professor emeritus at the Harvard Medical School, was a leader within the cure system in bringing together teams of surgeons, radiation therapists, chemotherapists, and pathologists to reevaluate treatment for breast cancer and to recognize the fallacy of thinking of cure in terms of five-year survival rate. Pertinent questions come up time after time. Does the treatment truly mitigate against the relentless course of the disease? Are there risks of introducing side effects even worse than the original disease? Does the prolongation of life have value for the patient? Are the choices understood, and is there help in reaching necessary decisions? As the number of days is extended, what will happen to the patient and family as a social unit? What will happen to them spiritually? When the possibility of cure is exhausted, how long should efforts to sustain and prolong life continue?

We must constantly take stock of what we know about palliative care and review advances in curative treatment to maintain a sound working relationship between the experts in each mode of care. The interweaving thread of "hospice care" for the patient with a terminal illness is a community of people who share tasks and resources, with a sense of total participation and collective decision-making. The dying, their families, and the caregivers form bonds seen in the respect they show one another. Intensity of involvement, anxiety provoked by embarking on unfamiliar territory, the necessity of making difficult decisions without sufficient evidence of balance between right and wrong, and the repeated experience of loss all create a situation where that respect is in a vulnerable position. It requires constant care to keep the working relationship in good order.

Edmund Pellegrino has said: "The whole unexplored territory of mutual obligation, mutual sharing of responsibility, and a requirement for a corporate sense of obligation in which each member of the team must feel responsibility for what his colleagues do or fail to do is put to the test." Home care hospice programs with clearly defined relationships to acute care hospitals offer services with a clear focus on strengthening community sources and resources. The opportunity of following the patient when he enters the hospital for specific treatment provides a continuity of care and the possibility of influencing the hospital's practices by demonstrating involvement with the patient and family to affirm their position as members of a community rather than their temporary relationships to a hospital. Hospice units within hospitals have a largely untapped capacity to change the very nature of hospital treatment. The essential humanism of hospice care, while offering patients, families, and staff a reciprocal system, is one aspect of emphasizing cure *and* care. Home care services are essential here, as well, along with the care of the family after the patient's death.

The nurse is the most likely professional to initiate a call to another agency or caregiver when a change in treatment is contemplated. Her skills in helping the family and patient to express what they want done, in providing all those involved with the information needed, in recognizing anxiety and in dealing with it can make or break the transition. If the health care system is to remain open so that the patient always has options in care throughout the illness, the nurse needs close collaboration with social worker, doctor, and the administrative assistant, but ultimately the nurse is responsible and accountable for meshing the links no matter how traditional, contemporary or avant garde a role she takes.

Reference

Henderson, V. 1966. *The Nature of Nursing: A Definition and Its Implications for Practice, Research, and Education*. New York: Macmillan.

16

Spiritual Care of the Dying Person

Steven A. Moss

Spiritual care is care of the inner person, the part of each human being created in God's image. The care of the inner person adds to his wholeness—it allows a human being to experience completeness in all aspects of his living and his dying. Not to enhance the inner person in everyone is to tarnish and detract from that sense of wholeness. Spiritual care is particularly important in our time of technological patient treatment and medical research because during such an era support of the whole person is often lacking. Such care can be provided optimally in a hospice; in fact, it is the very theme of hospice.

One of my patients, a 30-year-old woman, was suffering from breast cancer that had metastasized to the brain. As I visited on her floor and passed by her room, I could see her lying listlessly on the bed or sitting on the bed slumped over, her head almost touching her chest. She appeared to be in a deep sleep or in a stupor. Most staff members paid little or no attention to her. Assuming that she was either uninterested in or incapable of conversation, they would walk by her room and not even stop in to speak to her. Even when they were in her room to make her bed or deliver a tray, most staff ignored this woman.

Each time I walked into her room, I started a conversation. I would say "hello," and we would talk for a while about how she felt, who she was, and what she had done with her life. She always responded to my visits with warmth and interest. I discovered that she had a Master of Social Work degree. We talked about modern psychotherapeutic techniques, and I began to read psychology textbooks to her. Though the readings were not long, she found them meaningful and engaging. In time, I was even able to get her to play Scrabble with me. This was a significant accomplishment for this person who prior to my visits was assumed to be incapable of any communication and human interaction.

I related my experiences with her to other staff and members of her family. They began to realize that she was still a person with intellectual and emotional needs. She still possessed an inner person that felt, thought, and had hopes and dreams. The staff and family began to understand that she needed the feeling of "wholeness," of being treated as a person and not just as a disease and case number.

I shall never forget seeing her brother play Scrabble with her. This was someone who would not even enter his sister's room because he no longer saw her as one with needs he could fulfill. When he realized that she was still a person whose insides cried out for love, attention, and stimulation (which he could give), he was able to be with her and give of himself.

This experience demonstrates the difficulties present in caring for the terminally ill that a hospice strives to overcome. For this woman, as for so many other terminally ill persons, living in the face of dying becomes no life at all. The experience of life's end becomes

dying in an alien and sterile area, separated from the spiritual nourishment that comes from being able to reach out to a loving hand, separated from a desire to experience the things that make life worth living, separated from hope (Cousins 1979: 133).

It was not difficult for me to understand how death represented a goal of release for a patient I had visited. As she could look forward only to the pain of one operation after another, with no emotional and spiritual support from family and friends, she had nothing ahead of her but death itself. As her self-image had been destroyed, so too had her inner person.

How often terminal patients tell me that "this is no life." And for them it is not. They have lost a sense of security, a positive self-image, independence, self-worth, peace, wholeness, and personhood. No attention has been given to the inner person with its need to be treated physically, emotionally, spiritually, and intellectually. As one example, this woman whom I had visited had been left alone by staff and family, untouched in a human way by persons caring for her. Her physical needs were met, as were her medical needs. But her caregivers were unable to extend to her spiritual care by caring for and meeting the needs of her whole person. Once these inner needs had been met through communication with her by staff members and family, she could feel like a whole person and could face dying with more ease.

Often the terminally ill person is alienated from the living, isolated in a hospital or a chronic or nursing care facility, in which "the individual contracts his life process through isolation rather than [having] intensification of life through love..." (Beisheim 1972: 187). Care is usually not given beyond the objectified level of case history and case number. As Aries writes:

Death in the hospital is no longer the occasion of a ritual ceremony, over which the dying presides amidst his assembled relatives and friends. Death is a technical phenomenon obtained by a cessation determined in a more or less avowed way by decision of the doctor and the hospital team. Indeed, in the majority of cases the dying person has already lost consciousness.... Today the initiative has passed from the family, as much an outsider as the dying person, to the doctor and the hospital team. They are the masters of death. (1974: 18).

And even these "masters of death" stay away from the dying in the modern care facility. How often the surgeon ceases seeing a patient or visits only sporadically and briefly because that patient is terminal. As Parkes writes, "A busy surgical ward is not always a good place in which to die because staff are preoccupied with heroic efforts to save life and the patient who cannot be saved is a failure for all" (1972: 152).

How many nurses stay away from the dying patient so that he does not "die on her?" There are nurses who find that the "being-with" time demanded by the terminal patient is too emotionally draining. Such professionals consider patients who go home "well" less frustrating and destructive to their professional image. These staff attitudes make the patient feel like a nonperson, a "lung cancer" in the end bed, whose anxieties concerning dying then become heightened. Heightened anxieties lead to a more complicated physical, emotional, and spiritual picture and affect the dying process itself.

Alienation is enhanced by family and friends who, out of guilt, fear of open communication, or anticipatory grief, may withdraw from the patient.

The dying usually finds himself being abandoned as his condition deteriorates; the living have already "written him off." He becomes the central figure in a great "conspiracy of silence"—forbidden to voice his fears and lied to concerning his condition and progress (Kutscher and Goldberg 1973: 16).

I shall never forget the man dying of stomach cancer who lay in the bed before me bitter and upset as he told me that his wife was already dating other men. And what about family and friends hiding tearful eyes behind dark glasses, or not visiting at all out of fear of not knowing what to say or do, or not saying anything at all because of fright and fear? Again and again during my chaplaincy visits I am asked, "Why doesn't anyone come to see me?" If I were to answer, "Because you are dying," I would often be correct.

This kind of treatment for the dying is surely undesirable. In my opinion, time now dictates that society provide an atmosphere for the dying in which they are allowed to die with the sense of being a whole person. Spiritual care, as I have described it, must become operative for the dying.

An atmosphere must be provided for the terminal patient that gives support to him as a whole person, that provides a special warmth, genuine relationships, security, humane treatment, and respect. Whereas theoretically such an atmosphere could be created in any medical care institution, most are not able to introduce it. As a result, the hospice concept has been developing as a care system for the terminally ill.

All members of the hospice team are prepared to treat the patient as a person with a whole range of needs, dreams, and hopes, despite limited life expectancy.

The spiritual and psychological resources of the medical staff enable them to accept death as a meaningful event. . . in which the psychological as well as the physical needs of the patients are the central concern of everyone. [These resources] enable many patients in time to talk about the various fears and griefs that trouble them. . . . The disease is seen as one factor among many that influence the patient's peace of mind, attention is paid to the social climate. . . and physical and drug treatment is directed towards the relief of distressing symptoms. . . . Nurses know that they can sit and talk to patients without being told to get on with their work—talking to patients *is* [their] work (Parkes 1972: 152).

This hospice model creates a spiritual atmosphere where relationships are not I-It but are I-Thou, as they enhance the whole person. For families who participate in hospice, relationships with a dying loved one are enriched by open communication; and love and respect are fostered. The hospice staff is present to allow this to happen, to facilitate this kind of care, and to educate in this kind of caring.

What must be overcome in the care of the dying is the "progressive isolation and the development of a sense of 'aloneness'" (Feder 1976: 431). The hospice creates a social structure for the dying in which personal possessions, family and community, personal integrity, dignity, love, and comfort are allowed to be and to grow. Hospice takes holistic medicine, "treating the whole person in a system" (Black 1980: 213), and applies it to care of the dying. This is the underlying spiritual care for the terminally ill that is the basic philosophy of hospice. It has been written of hospice:

They can offer, instead of mechanical resuscitation, a hospitable place in which the personal and spiritual growth of the individual can continue during the process of dying. . . . [Patients] need life around them, spiritual and emotional comfort and support of every sort. . . . They need their own clothes, their own pictures, music, food, surroundings that are familiar to them, people they know and love, people they can trust to care about them (Stoddard 1978: 28, 67-68).

References

Aries, P. 1974. *Western Attitudes Toward Death: From the Middle Ages to the Present*. Baltimore: The Johns Hopkins University Press.

Beisheim, P. 1972. "Death and Dying: Life and Living." In G. Devine, ed., *That They May Live: Theological Reflections on the Quality of Life*. New York: Alba House.

Black, D. 1980. "Medicine and the Mind." *Playboy* 27 (4).

Cousins, N. 1979. *Anatomy of an Illness as Perceived by the Patient*. New York: W. W. Norton.

Feder, S. 1976. "Attitudes of Patients with Advanced Malignancy." In E. Shneidman, ed., *Death: Current Perspectives*. New York: Jason Aronson.

Kutscher, A. H. and M. R. Goldberg, eds. 1973. *Caring for the Dying Patient and His Family*. New York: Health Sciences Publishing Co.

Parkes, C. M. 1972. *Bereavement*. New York: International Universities Press.

Stoddard, S. 1978. *The Hospice Movement*. New York: Vintage Books.

17

Death Is Not All at Once ...Living Is Day By Day

Luis F. Martorell

As a social worker practitioner in private practice, I have worked for many years with dying patients in their own homes. I am not a member of a hospice team, but I am aware of the needs of the dying patient and his family for more specialized psychological help in coping with the stresses of a terminal illness. With the development of the hospice movement in the United States efforts have been directed toward giving this help in the dying patient's home. My initial therapeutic contact takes place in the home and my major concern is helping the family to cope with the crisis of terminal illness.

During the first family visit, I assess the family and their situation by looking at how they communicate, their strengths and weaknesses, what resources they have, and what they need from the community and others. I encourage the family to establish immediate goals about their manner of relating to each other and living through this period. I explain the importance and benefits to be derived from home visits rather than from office visits. Usually, I visit the home once a week but increase or decrease visits according to the family's needs.

Home visits give the worker direct contact with the daily living of the family. By the nature of the setting, office visits establish and maintain a certain distance between worker and family. Seeing the patient and his family in their own environment leads to a more trusting and intimate relationship. The worker is able to observe the normal interacting of the patient and his family, and this is a very important factor during this crisis period. For example, the worker gets to know the family culture, values, beliefs, and philosophies. As the worker becomes more involved with the family, he comes to be considered a part of the family. At this point, it is necessary to avoid making decisions for the family. It is imperative then for him to maintain his role as a resource at hand who is able and willing to help the family members to deal with themselves and to arrive at their own decisions.

I have realized the paradox of the coexistence of living and dying as it affects each family member. To some extent, the healthy and the dying are both involved in these two processes. The family is involved in the dying process of the patient because a part of each of them is dying. Similarly, the patient is in the living process that continues until his death. In the beginning some members of the family may deny the imminent death of the loved one and the effect it is having on all of them, but the worker must help them face it before the actual death occurs. This denial is evidence that the family is not experiencing anticipatory grief, a necessary and beneficial process for helping the dying patient cope with his own death. The process of anticipatory grief also helps the family members with the stresses of everyday living.

Anticipatory grief (Aldrich 1974) describes the grief process occurring before a loss. The grief experienced by the dying patient must occur in anticipation of losing everything—spouse, home, family, job, position. On the other hand, the family faces the stage of anticipating loss, as well as the stage of the reality of loss that follows the death. When the family engages in anticipatory grieving, the grieving process that follows death is shortened.

It is necessary for the worker to break through any denial that is blocking the anticipatory process in both family and patient. When the patient and family begin to deal with anticipatory grief, an opportunity to establish and reinforce stronger relationships in a stressful situation is created. Recognition of feelings for each other that have never been expressed may surface, be verbalized, and handled in a more positive way. The period of anticipatory grieving also has a negative side, a hostile component of ambivalence and opportunity for destructive potential. While a long period of anticipation can increase the destructive potential, it also offers more time for working through the problems.

When a dying patient is treated in the home, the worker must be aware of emergencies. He should be prepared to handle them when there are no other team members to help the family. Joe, a sixty-five-year-old man, was dying of cancer and emphysema. I became aware that he was extremely angry and that most of his anger was displaced on his 13-year-old son Keith. This displacement of anger became so extreme that it disrupted the family. Following emergency telephone calls from Joe's wife, I made a drop-in visit. The family was in tremendous turmoil. Everyone except the dying patient was in the living room. The mother was crying, and it was obvious that Keith was very frightened although he was camouflaging this with anger. I told the family I would see Joe first. Joe, who could breathe only with the use of an oxygen mask (and even then it was a noisy, painful process), had the oxygen turned up as high as possible. He was angry and breathing with such difficulty that his speaking voice was unclear. Joe felt he could no longer tolerate Keith. He accused him of constantly coming into his room to harass him with questions. After Joe had expressed his anger, I helped him understand that it was directed more toward his incapacitation than toward Keith. As we talked, Joe began to realize that he had a tremendous fear of suffocating to death. Every time he became upset with Keith, breathing became more distressed; subconsciously he began to anticipate increased difficulty in breathing whenever Keith came in.

It took almost two hours for Joe to calm down. He welcomed my suggestion that a plan of action be taken such as making a contract with Keith to control behavior that was anger provoking to his father. I then involved the mother and the two teenage children in an emergency session. All three finally ventilated the fear that the father was going to die. For the first time his imminent death became a reality to them, and they were able to talk with emotion about it. I then explained to Keith that his behavior was caused by his own fears that if he was not with his father, Joe might die. It seemed obvious that Keith's method of provoking anger was his own way of keeping his father alive. I suggested a contract for Keith whereby he agreed to be with his father only twice daily for five to ten minutes.

In subsequent visits, I learned that father and son were getting along much better, and communication among the family was much improved. If I had failed to respond to the emergency needs of Joe and his family, it is conceivable that Joe's extreme emotion that night could have interfered with his breathing until he suffocated. If his death had occurred in this way, it would have left the family, especially Keith, with a terrible burden of guilt.

I hope to help the patient maintain and exercise his rights and maintain his dignity. The patient has the right to grieve for his own death and the right to know as much as he wants about his illness and treatment. Sometimes the patient is afraid to exercise this right, and the worker needs to make him aware of his fear and help him overcome it. A Catholic brother was dying of cancer. After he returned from the hospital to the community home where he lived with 23 members of his community, I began to visit him two or three times a week. On one of these visits I realized that he was extremely depressed. In talking I discovered that the depression was mainly the result of his not knowing the extent of his illness. As a result of a religious background where obedience was emphasized, he felt that he was not "worthy" of demanding a better explanation of his illness and treatment from his doctor. It took several intensive sessions before he could accept that he had that right.

The fact that a dying patient is in his own home with his family does not in itself mean that he still retains his same position or feels a part of the family. The level and quality of communication connect him with his family. There are three possibilities of communication that may take place. First, the family might avoid communication and thus make the patient feel completely isolated or even cause members of the family to become isolated from each other, as well as from the dying patient.

On another occasion with the Catholic brother, his depression was the result of a "conspiracy of silence" that his 23 brothers were unconsciously subjecting him to by avoiding him. One of his close friends informed me of how isolated the patient felt. I decided that "manipulation of the environment" would be the most effective means of handling the situation. I had two sessions with the 23 brothers in which I explained the process of dying so that they would understand what the patient was going through. They had avoided the dying brother because his dying made them very uncomfortable. They did not know how to relate to him. In the second session, an interactional group helped them verbalize and face their own fears about death. In a subsequent visit I noticed that the "family" began to spend time with the dying patient. Toward the end, this patient went to a nursing home where he had specialized care. All of the brothers were able to visit him.

A second possibility with communication is that the family can interact socially and yet carefully avoid any talk of impending death. In this case denial is blocking the anticipatory grief. As a worker I handle this kind of denial with a diversity of techniques such as role playing, Gestalt, or Transactional Analysis. In one instance with a black family, the patient's wife was the only family member denying the imminent death of her husband. I discovered in family sessions that she had never really grieved for her father's death, which had occurred four or five years previously. Through the use of Gestalt techniques she realized she had never accepted her father's death. After accepting and grieving for her father's death, she was able to realistically face the approaching death of her husband.

The third (and ideal) possibility with communication occurs when the family member and the dying patient respond naturally and openly to the needs and feelings of each other. This implies a continuation of normal, appropriate human responses to what is happening now that death has entered the picture. It is unfortunate that our social mores have not prepared us for an easy, flowing movement into the ideal form of communication where death is concerned. Professional help is often required for the family to achieve this desirable, more free communication.

It is extremely important to help the family and dying patient recognize and complete as much unfinished business as possible. This will greatly reduce the weight of the post-death grieving of the family and will reduce their burden of guilt, anxiety, and remorse. This helps the relationship and is a part of the anticipatory grieving process done directly with the patient while he is alive. It facilitates the dying process for the patient and permits him to live more fully in the time he has left.

During anticipatory grieving the worker helps patient and family face what will happen to the family in the future. Inclusion of the patient in these discussions will give the patient the feeling that the family is giving him permission to die. I have experienced a dying patient's satisfaction when he has been a part of discussions about family restructure, change in roles, members' responsibilities, and the possibilities of working out new philosophies. The dying patient feels he is more in charge of his life, and it is easier for him to give and receive love and care.

Reference

Aldrich, C. K. 1974. "Some Dynamics of Anticipatory Grief." In B. Schoenberg et al., eds., *Anticipatory Grief*, pp. 3—9. New York: Columbia University Press.

18

The Role of a Clinical Psychologist

Arthur C. Carr

The role of a clinical psychologist on a service for terminal patients should be accepted as an obvious and routine one. Unfortunately, this is not always so. Other professionals, such as nurses, social workers, activity and recreational therapists, and clergy, offer functions and skills that are readily acknowledged as relevant to the care of physically ill and dying patients, as well as to their families. Nevertheless, the clinical psychologist might have to make his own defense for what he has to offer in a setting that in most instances is primarily medically oriented and geared to physical management of the patient, where the assumption is that the presence of medicine both as a profession and as an elixir is what really matters most.

In an effort to discern what the clinical psychologist could offer in a setting specifically planned for preterminal and terminal patients, it might be helpful to review briefly the qualifying educational and training experiences generally required in today's university doctoral programs. The graduate programs in clinical psychology are more formalized than for psychology students with other majors, since approval of such programs by the American Psychological Association requires adherence to broad general outlines and principles deemed basic to any adequate training program for clinical psychologists.

Prerequisites

a) An undergraduate college degree (usually B.A. or B.S.) that has included a broad range of subjects, covering both the social and physical sciences;

b) elementary courses in experimental design, introductory psychology, abnormal psychology, personality theory, and statistics that are usually also considered mandatory;

c) a minimum of three academic years of full-time graduate study;

d) instruction in scientific and professional ethics, research design, statistics, and psychometrics;

e) competence in substantive content areas of the biological bases of behavior (generally covered by courses in physiological psychology, neuropsychology, sensation and perception, psychopharmacology), cognitive-affective bases of behavior (covered by courses in learning, motivation, emotion), social bases of behavior (covered by courses in social psychology, group processes, systems theory), and individual differences (covered by courses in personality theory, human development, psychopathology);

f) supervised practicums and field experiences, culminating in a full-time, one-year internship to provide clinical experience appropriate to the area of specialty;

g) a written dissertation usually involving an original research project designed and executed by the student, deemed to be one that makes a substantial contribution to the knowledge in the field.

The total graduate program usually requires four to five years beyond the undergraduate degree. To qualify then for the National Register of Health Service Providers in Psychology, the clinical psychologist, in addition to having a doctorate degree in psychology from a regionally accredited university, must also be licensed or certified at the independent practice level by a state board of examiners in psychology and also have two years of supervised experience in psychology, of which one year must be postdoctoral.

Competition today for better doctoral programs in clinical psychology is possibly greater than that for most medical schools, and it is definitely just as great. Difficult as some psychiatrists may find it to believe, applicants today are not persons who, for some reason, "could not make it" to medical school. Evidence indicates that present applicants are individuals highly motivated to the study of human behavior, that is, *psychology*, viewing it as a science and a profession quite apart from medicine and its preoccupation with disease, presenting intellectual challenges and rewards that exceed those they view as emanating from the study of medicine.

Thus, the clinical psychologist comes with a background unlike that of any other professional and should be able to make a unique contribution to any setting that deals with preterminal or terminally ill patients. In my opinion, the clinical psychologist might have significant impact in many different areas.

The clinical psychologist comes with special abilities in conceptualizing and executing research designs. It does appear that the area of research in thanatology has not moved forward aggressively. Certainly, more than a decade ago, when the Foundation of Thanatology was being conceived, I anticipated that by this time there would be available much more hard-core data from across the country than seems to be the case. It is with disappointment that one must state that the best available research data in thanatology—and perhaps even the best models for care of the terminally ill patient—have come from other countries, particularly England, Canada, and Australia. A defensive argument for this could be based on the facts that the hospice involvement itself originated in Great Britain and that governmental funding supported its innovative programs.

A simple example of a researchable question is that involving where the most suitable place to die is, not only in terms of the comfort and physical well-being of the patient, but also in terms of the short-term and long-term effects on the bereaved. With a philosophy somewhat akin to that of Woody Allen, who states that he knows he's going to die—it's just that he just doesn't want to be around when it happens—it is my impression that there is a tendency today to overromanticize the notion of "dying at home." If so, I presume this tendency was based, to some degree, on the finding by Rees and Lutkins (1967) that in England the risk of close relatives' dying during the first year of bereavement was significantly greater when the death causing the bereavement had occurred some place other than at home. But this one example in the area of grief and my knowledge of the bereavement practices in England— particularly in those sections that from our standpoint would be considered rural—raise a question of whether death in the home might not have entirely different implications than in a crowded Manhattan apartment where the bed or bedroom of the deceased may be needed badly enough so as to require its use the first night after the death has occurred. While we may think of guilt's being generated by one's absence from the scene when a loved one dies, there are other emotions—revulsion, fear, horror—that may be accentuated in children (and even adults) who must continue living in the same setting in which a death has just occurred. I do not suggest that this is inevitable, but it is one of the legitimate issues that could be better investigated. To assume that there is something especially commendable about dying at home, while disparaging what has been labeled the "white, sterile atmosphere of a hospital," might not be entirely justified, at least in all situations or with all illnesses.

There has been too much ready acceptance of folklore and personal impressions in thanatology. How readily the Elizabeth Kübler-Ross' "stages of dying" were accepted as gospel, even though they did not conform to our own experience! How readily the notion that terminally ill patients always know or always should know (be told) that they are dying also seemed to become part of a dogmatic "package." In a time when open communication—letting it all "hang out"—is being taken for granted in relation to sex, it is easy to assume that a similar attitude about death and dying should necessarily apply. Certainly we have seen that some individuals have made a well-publicized career out of their own terminal illnesses. Certainly about many we can only feel, as was said about Cawdor—that "Nothing in their lives became them like the leaving it." But do we not know that different personality types use quite different types of defenses and coping methods? Is denial necessarily the *worst* defense that one can use? Might it not even be the only one to provide support for a patient? When does denial work adequately and when doesn't it? Does a model derived essentially from work with cancer patients apply equally to all other illnesses? And how does one know? Evangelical discourses on "dying with dignity" do not tell! With training in the study of individual differences, the clinical psychologist should be able to elucidate relevant patient variables.

Because the psychologist has had special emphasis in his training on what constitutes "truth"—I must add quickly, only in terms of interpretation of statistical probability values of an experiment—it seems to me that he might be the best professional to have around to help order situations, observations on them, and conclusions about them, since most other professionals may be too burdened with the immediate clinical needs in the situation to worry much about "generalizability of findings."

I suspect sophistication about research design has made most psychologists aware of the possible influence of factors that may seem peripheral to others. More aware of experimental variables, the psychologist, for example, in general, might become concerned with the visual impact of any ward or unit being planned for the care of the terminally ill. When do planned facilities designed to foster interpersonal intimacy lead only to the effects of overcrowding? What are ideal space requirements in a setting for terminal patients? What are the psychological effects of color and lighting?

I have long had the personal hunch—not substantiated by research—that physicians, particularly psychiatrists as a group, tend to be primarily auditory individuals, while the psychologists I have known tend to be primarily visual. No pejorative judgment is implied, but at least this is how I explain the fact that physicians are considered the professional group who contribute most to the Metropolitan Opera, something I think cannot be accounted for solely on the grounds of income level. It is also how I explain what seems sometimes to be the physicians' willingness and ability to tolerate such dreary and depressing physical working conditions, seemingly never questioning whether their work environment must be as visually unappealing as it usually is.

Obviously, my hunch, even if true, does not account for the whole picture. Undoubtedly the advent of the antibiotics greatly changed the rules about what priorities the physician represented and valued. Good nursing care, rest, nourishing food, fresh air, open space, sunlight, time spent listening to the patient—sometimes the main or only ingredients to patient care in bygone days—became less important than penicillin in the patient's recovery to many now readily curable disorders. The bedside manner of a kindly, lovable white-headed gentleman in a white coat really did become less important. The surgeon may indeed be a tyrant—we do not prefer surgeons of this type, of course—but if the choice is between lovability and surgical competence, we know what to opt for! Nevertheless, when surgery and other medical advances are no longer relevant to the care of a dying patient, we may find it advantageous to recall what constituted ideal care in bygone days.

The clinical psychologist on a terminal facility should also help explicate not only crucial subject (i.e., patient) variables and environmental (i.e., facility) variables but also experimenter variables (i.e., those related to the staff). Working on such a facility is undoubtedly one of the most stressful jobs, where it can be presumed that many of the personnel are brought together because of their own unique experiences with loss and bereavement and harbor the underlying wish for a catharsis and a release from the past. Becoming disillusioned or "burnt-out" will be common reactions. In such a setting, opportunities for staff conflict, both latent and overt, will be great. It is generally less painful to be angry than to be depressed; avoidance of intimacy is often a defense against fully experiencing either emotion. With awareness of group processes, the clinical psychologist would offer skills in group therapy and conflict resolution in a setting where projection and denial are too easily generated. To be studied and documented is the effect of unresolved staff disagreement (and its subsequent resolution) on patient disease, since we already know how, in a psychiatric setting, at least, patient acting-out is often a response to unresolved staff differences and is found to diminish when such differences are resolved in conference.

Biomedical advances that sometimes grow directly out of medicine's new capabilities in preserving life have raised many value and ethical questions that are not easily answered. Such questions, it seems to me, will multiply in the future and will be especially relevant in a setting where patients are, by definition, labeled preterminal or terminal. Consider, for example, the complexity of the issues that might arise with a patient, considered terminal for one illness, who now develops another illness that may or may not itself be terminal. How actively should treatment of the latter be pursued particularly if resources are limited? Is the second illness possibly a "blessing"? Supposing the treatments for the two illnesses are incompatible? Which specialist prevails? How are these and attending questions to be resolved? Here, I would hope that a clinical psychologist, as a nonmedical professional, might offer fresh viewpoints or at least approaches to arriving at them. Are not ethical and value questions simply too important to be left in the hands of physicians and clergy? Isn't it unfair to expect these professionals to have the unshared burden of many such decisions?

With skills related to research, teaching, and service, including both psychological diagnosis and treatment, the clinical psychologist, I would think, should find a busy, productive career on a continuing care service. I think he would soon prove himself indispensable.

Obviously, the character of whom I speak should ideally have more than the formal training qualifications I reported. I would hope the clinical psychologist had qualities generally not even considered in standard psychological or psychiatric evaluations, qualities I hope other staff personnel also had: courage, sense of humor, commitment, humility, willingness to respect fully the patient's religious beliefs, and, finally, a continuing recognition that, in the final analysis—whether ill or well, young or old, doctor or patient—"We are all," in Sullivan's words, "much more simply human than otherwise."

Reference

Rees, W. D. and S. G. Lutkins. 1967. "Mortality of Bereavement." *British Medical Journal* 4: 13ff.

19

Group Therapy for Life Enrichment

Sharon McMahon

What does death mean to you? To some people, it's the "grand perhaps." To others it's the "poor man's doctor." To still others, it's punishment... relief... unfair ... the grand leveler ... merciful ... eternal sleep ... terrifying, a delightful hiding place for weary men.

To some, death is the "new pornography"—a subject hidden from today's children and not discussed openly among adults, even professionals. Indeed, few among us like to think about the subject. And yet, nurses in particular, must. As a comforting companion to people on their way to face death, nurses are often more apt to witness death than perhaps almost any group—except perhaps soldiers in wartime. ("Probe," *Nursing' 74*, p. 59.)

There are counselors, hospital chaplains, and thanatologists endeavoring to enrich lives and to comfort and counsel the dying, their significant others, and the staff responsible for their medical care.

Pincus states:

Thinking and talking about death need not be morbid; they may be quite the opposite. Ignorance and fear of death overshadow life, while knowing about and accepting death erases his shadow and makes life freer of fears and anxieties. The fuller and richer people's experience of life the less death seems to matter to them—as if love of life casts out fear of death. A child therapist once said to me, "Children of parents who are not afraid of death are not afraid of life." In that sense, education for death is education for life, and should be an underlying feature in all education in schools, universities, and through the media. (Pincus 1976: 250)

The life crisis of death and the dying–grieving continuum has, to this time, been a private and often lonely period, not openly exposed to the action and social influences of preparatory group discussion and therapy. Curran states: "Resistance to the limits of the human condition seems so basic that it tends to keep us intellectualized rather than allowing us to enter into genuine and personal engagement with life in ourselves or others."

This resistance to the termination and vulnerability of human life makes it difficult for man to think of his life as finite. Curran continues:

Man does not wish to subject himself to total human experience as it really is. If he actually submits to it, he does so with resistance, even hostility. Man takes a risk and chances failure and self-defeat if he lets himself experience his finite condition. The contradiction in this, however, is that he has no real sense of personal value and achievement unless he does so. Personal redemption—in the meaning of having acquired a sense of one's personal value and worth—only follows upon personal incarnation (Curran 1972: 67).

Efforts toward submission to the human experience, toward attempts to find meaning in life and personal incarnation can validate an individual's worth to self and others. The author proposes that counseling as a means of increasing life's meaning and feelings of self-worth can facilitate these efforts. Explored in this paper are the effects of group therapy in a palliative care unit where chronically ill dying patients seek a peaceful, dignified end in death.

Approaches

Kübler-Ross, a missionary of the new meanings and approaches to death and dying, notes:

...it is evident that the terminally ill patient has very special needs which can be fulfilled if we take the time to sit and listen and find out what they are. The most important communication, perhaps, is the fact that we let him know that we are ready and willing to share some of his concerns. To work with the dying patient requires a certain maturity which only comes from experience. We have to take a good hard look at our own attitude toward death and dying before we can sit quietly without anxiety next to a terminally ill patient (Kübler-Ross 1969: 269).

This challenge confronts the group leader working with the individual feelings, needs, and life priorities of those who can no longer deny or resist the portent of death and finiteness of their physical beings. New approaches are being developed throughout the world (Feifel 1977) to support the continuance of family life, personal growth, and living, while the inevitability of death flows into the therapeutic plan. Ontario has the Victorian Order of Nurses, Homemakers Services and Physicians who make home care possible while psychological and spiritual aspects of self are cared for through specially trained counselors and pastors.

When patients enter the hospital, they leave their own community and much of their identity. We are all bound up in our homes and our possessions, our work and our hobbies, and we feel stripped and humiliated if our clothes and personal belongings are removed. The emphasis on possessions, clothes, and idiosyncracies in a hospice is a way of maintaining identity. Many hospital wards do little to integrate their patients into a new community in which they have an active part.

People matter more than things, and a patient is, above all, part of a family and circle of friends. St. Christopher's Hospice (London) tries to welcome the family as wholeheartedly as it greets the patient who is part of it (Feifel 1977: 168).

A study by Parkes (1975) states that when unsupported families were visited twenty months after bereavement, they were found to have twice as much depression as "supported" families. They also had significantly more physical symptoms of anxiety (Feifel: 170). Could group therapy help reduce these symptoms of maladjustment to their loss?

According to Pinkel,

If it becomes apparent that the child in relapse will not regain remission status, it is important to formulate with the family plans for terminal care. For many families the death of the child is better conducted at home or in a community hospital. Most families and patients accept death courageously if they have had ample opportunity to discuss their feelings with each other and with a trusted physician throughout the course of the disease (Pinkel 1976: 128).

With the help of society and counselors on the health team, therapy groups could be made a common, voluntary part of the dying process.

Process

Feifel suggests: "It has been said that a society consists of those who are united in the service of a common purpose, focusing first and foremost on the work to be done together" (1977: 176).

In helping those with terminal illness,

much of the weariness and mental suffering may still remain, but it is deeply rewarding to meet people who are making such achievements of life's pattern and to join in such occasions. We cannot take away the whole hard thing that is happening, but celebration is still an important part of life, and each hospice occasion is a salute to this kind of courage. There is no need for the staff to idealize their patients, the daily reality of troubles accepted and overcome is enough. Neither patients, families, nor staff are protected from sadness, but in sharing it as they do they find that living and dying well are linked together and are constantly opening up new and creative possibilities (1977: 177).

Feifel continues that there are process steps within the environment of a hospice or palliative care unit that can serve as a basis for group selection, task development, and interventions by a counselor with patients, staff, and families. These are informed consent, safe conduct, significant survival, anticipatory grief, timeliness, and appropriate death (1977: 45). One final consideration, that of "pragnanz" (Banet 1974: 182) or readiness, is needed before implementing the group process with members who share the common "contextual elements" (p. 181) critical to the phenomena of death, dying, and mourning.

Objectives

Banet states further that: "Psychotherapeutic objectives are often vague because few people come to psychotherapy with a clearly stated objective (1974: 182)." It is therefore meaningful for the counselor to meet individually with clients to allow each one to develop their personal goals for membership and participation. The leader must also have some self-awareness, goal direction, and basic objectives to keep the group process mobilized.

Listed below are possible objectives for groups dealing with such circumstances as personal death; loss of a family member; loss of body image, by amputation, abortion, or miscarriage; personal feelings when caring for dying patients/clients; and life support by mechanical means.

a) To be able to give honest answers to children, adolescents, and adults appropriate for their conceptions, development, understanding, and anxiety;

b) to understand loss of control, fear of separation and the dark, loneliness, anomie, meaninglessness, and pain as personal behavioral responses;

c) to be aware of, understand, and accept the physiological changes related to dying and mourning depressions;

d) to promote the presence of familiar objects, pets, and people in a palliative setting;

e) to encourage "normal" attachment activities such as giving and receiving love from significant people (lover, spouse, parents, siblings) in the client's life, and increase "availability" of staff (Schmidt 1972: 1087);

f) to prevent detachment and regression due to unresolved conflicts and dishonest, unrealistic relationships;

g) to emphasize the importance and preference of home care;

h) to encourage exploration of feelings, attitudes, beliefs, values, and traditions related to self, life, death, rituals, and after life;

i) to keep open lines of communication of all types—attending, listening, symbols, touch, verbalization, singing, presence;

j) to explore the implications and impact of death on the family unit in terms of (leadership, social changes, cultural concomitants, financial and legal pressures, cognitive and emotional factors) and to protect vulnerable members during "crisis" periods;

k) to demonstrate skills and to reduce pain, disruptions, mutilation, isolation and promote rest, orderliness, stimulation, comfort, dignity, and human trust, contact, and love and thereby increase the competence of staff and family members;

l) to explore the nature of personal adjustments to death and preparation for saying goodbye;

m) to develop awareness of stages of grief, anger, guilt, symptom formation, depression, relief, and adjustment;

n) to encourage use of community resources as supportive groups for mental health;

o) to construct activities in which concerns, thoughts, feelings, and magical fantasies can be safely ventilated and distortions corrected;

p) to promote realistic, consistent feedback from environment, people, and self;

q) to encourage honest faith and genuine respect;

r) to educate people in the modalities of maintenance and therapeutic and palliative care;

s) to complete funeral/cremation plans and disbursements of goods;

t) to prepare family for distortions in time, sensations, and ability to concentrate; fears of being alone in the house; anorexia and/or insomnia; loss of meaning in life; loss of desire to accept responsibility; "paranoid" reactions of a temporary nature;

u) to establish phone contact with others in the group to act as a crisis link;

v) to establish and restore equilibrium for mourners.

Conflicts

McElroy (1975: 26) discusses the care of the untreated infant and states that in some large institutions, "the attending staff reach a point in the treatment of a child when it becomes physically and morally necessary to 'back off'—to terminate active and aggressive care for the child." It is essential for staff and parents to get together to explore personal and professional feelings, life potential, legal implications, resources, and stressors related to this child's (and even an adult's) care. They must grapple with the question posed by McElroy: "At what point does one lose or gain the right to die with purpose, dignity and consideration" (p. 30)?

The group leader must be aware of his personal objectives, feelings, beliefs, and maturity level in working with the dying person of any age. As feelings and responses tend to differ with the person's age, disease, and form of "chronicity" or acuteness of death, ethical and moral responses may not be consistent.

Communication

Brill describes three basic modes of communication—verbal, nonverbal, and symbolic. These can be given and received at various levels as Berne (in Brill 1973: 43) theorized and applied in his transactional analysis model of individual and group therapy.

Perception of community is influenced by the cultural background and present life experiences of the perceiver. Cultural variations can create barriers to effective communication and perception. It is important, therefore, to clarify the messages and determine their meaning to sender and receiver and observers in the setting.

Story telling, words, movements and posture, dress and grooming, pictures, music, humor, writings, food, gifts, time together, body distance, and facial expression are all significant modes of communication between the dying person, caregivers, family, friends, and others and must be clarifed or responded to to promote clarity, awareness, and insight and prevent assumptions, lost meanings, and confusion.

One of the most potent and universal methods of communication is touch. Northrup (1974: 1068) suggests that "touch—holding a parent's (person's) hand or putting a gentle arm around someone's shoulders— frequently narrows the distance between the family (and others), and creates a supportive bond between them." Therefore, a group leader need not fear "touch" as a mode to support (or substitute for) verbalization, listening, intellectualization, rehearsing, and sharing in therapeutic groups (Williams 1976: 55; Drummond 1970: 57-59).

Barriers

In many ways all the aspirations, objectives, and techniques are not easily applied to the therapeutic realm of the dying and mourning. Resistance or denial is often seen in adults and adolescents who refuse to acknowledge the idea of death, not to mention the reality of its influence upon their lives. Children do not deny death but rather fantasize their power to control it (Kopp 1975: 1).

Other adults act out their childhood struggles and limited self-esteem when death threatens them. "I've been cheated of my life. I won't stand for it. I must have my own way, if not earlier, then now. Others won't be able to get their way with me, or use me ever again."

Adults reproach themselves, force others to feel sorry for them, and demand love. If love is not forthcoming, they will bully, bribe, sulk, upset others, be "sneaky" and bad enough to obtain their own way—or give up.

Kopp states that part of the therapist's role is to avoid getting entangled by the "patient's attempts at emotional blackmail, intimidation, seduction, adoration, dependent demands, and the like." The leader should attempt to arouse the client's interest in life. The self-disrupting and defeating activities may be analyzed and must be stopped. Feelings and empathic responses must be given to let the patient know that he is as valuable a person as he wants to believe he really is.

In the following anecdote Mr. J., a patient with a highly malignant brain tumor, has just joined the spontaneously formed "feelings sharing session" in the lounge.

"I have more pain than any of you. My tears are bitter and may scars are permanent. I have so much to lose—all I have, all we have. My loneliness for my Anna is so aching in my chest that I cannot breathe. Who are you—any of you—to think and feel you have any more to lose? I live in the same imperfect, hellish world. I have to make do with much less than I want—than I wish or shall ever have."

Another member says, "You make me angry, even sick! Do you think you are any worse off than any of the others of us—than me? I too want to succeed, to win, to love without loss, to reach out without risk." Harsh glares are exchanged.

Therapist: "Welcome to the club. While the rest of us are listening, we feel we must sometimes fall, feel foolish or inadequate, but we rise again and go on. Why do you, Mr. J., feel you alone should be spared all this?" Discussion opens and feelings and reflections are shared.

According to Kopp (p. 3), it is important for the leader to help each group member to see "that for each of them this session is an hour of his life, no more to be recaptured by the one than by the other. They could become important to one another, but only to the extent that each disarms himself, takes chances on being vulnerable to be hurt by the other, to risk new losses." Group members must be encouraged to "unhook from the past to make do with the rest of the world" (Kopp, p. 3).

It is the action of mourning that helps in the normal restorative process. These reactions can be related to shock and disbelief of anger and hostility of dying and death. Crying and tears "often takes place during the second phase—developing awareness. Because tears are important to the process of normal grieving, they should not be discouraged and should be allowed to continue" (Ren Kneisl 1976: 39).

Leadership

Johnson and Johnson (1975: 23) express the theory of functional leadership in two basic ideas: "(1) any member of a group may become a leader by taking actions that serve group functions, and (2) any leadership function may be fulfilled by different members performing a variety of revelant behaviors."

The task maintenance roles of the organizing leader may be carried on, but the leadership style should be flexible enough to motivate and encourage members to take on leadership. However, with decreasing desire to take on responsibility, the leader may find group members less willing to take leadership for even a short time.

Sharing and helping others with experiences to increase awareness and acceptance of death in others may be one motivating factor that will encourage group cohesion. Other functions of the therapeutic leader are "encourager, harmonizer, compromiser, tension reliever, energizer, communication helper, evaluator, process observer, standard setter, reality tester, summarizer, active listener, trust builder, and inter-personal problem solver" (Johnson and Johnson 1975: 28).

Before groups can effectively deal with group problems, they must trust others and themselves. This basic developmental stage can be an excellent foundation upon which to build therapeutic communication. The level of personal and group trust could be evaluated within the group, before and after experiences. This is important to improve the effectiveness of the group. Trust can be evaluated by using the following model (Johnson and Johnson 1975: 244).

	High Acceptance, Support, and Cooperative Intentions	*Low Acceptance, Support, and Cooperative Intentions*
High Openness and Sharing:	Trusting and trustworthy	Trusting but untrustworthy
Low Openness and Sharing:	Distrustful but trustworthy	Distrustful and untrustworthy

The group leader may be responsible for establishing the level of trust by acting as a role model and honestly sharing personal experiences, feelings, and reactions with members.

Do and Do Not

Beachy helped with the principles of group process and conduction by developing a list of do's and don'ts related to the dying and grieving:

Do Not	Do
try to whitewash the difficulty of pain, suffering, death, human failure, and misunderstanding;	face fully the facts of pain, suffering, death, human failure, and misunderstanding, by doing all that is possible to overcome them;
be cold to human grief or unaccepting of the emotional reactions of those who are hurt;	rise to the challenge of surmounting your own faults and have faith in all persons to do the same;
become defensive when at fault, either by denying or downgrading the responsibility, or by seeking too eagerly for expressions of understanding and acceptance;	have more concern for the welfare of the bereaved than for the protection of the institution;
give the impression of withholding information or hiding facts;	depend upon the strength of good relationships with the doctor, the nurse, the chaplain, and others to be a healing influence;
become impatient with the time required to obtain an adequate response or otherwise lose control of your own emotions;	make it possible at the right time for the family to become aware of the precautions taken to avoid accidents and the vigilance exercised to reduce them;
wait for the occurrence of such an event to prepare to meet it, or neglect anything which may be done to assure maximum preparation;	remember that the process of adjustment lasts longer than the brief period after death when hospital personnel are with the family. Continue communication through openness to further questions, availability of later reports, and personal attention of high-echelon personnel to final practical details;
mistakenly conceive that communication is all verbal or that only what is communicated at the time is applicable;	
be oversolicitous;	expand the area of help by fostering the continued care and attention of a clergyman or other supportive person;

All have significance for grief counselors who are helping people to unhook from the ties of living and to establish a firm trust in self and in the meaning of life.

Leader Guidelines

Guidelines for personal involvement must be drawn up to promote facilitative, flexible group leadership. Kavanaugh (1976) suggests:

a) Define your role as advocate and informant.
b) Maintain an abiding respect for your own personal needs.
c) Understand and respect the unique grieving process as it unfolds within yourself and within all those even peripherally involved.
d) Find ways of dealing with institutional grief.
e) Take a break or ask for a temporary transfer when you reach your emotional limits.
f) Be, as best you can, the kind of person whose presence bespeaks acceptance and nonjudgment.
g) No medical or moral law prevents secrets between adult and child.
h) You can easily enter a child's world without loss of dignity or propriety if you respond to him from the child within yourself.
i) Forget not the parents or families who need privacy to work out shock and disorganization.

Growth Group

Most growth-group experiences involve interpersonal skills of (1) initiating, building, and maintaining relationships with other people that are fulfilling and trusting (this skill includes self disclosure, giving and receiving feedback, trust and self-acceptance); (2) communicating ideas and feelings correctly, unambiguously verbally and nonverbally; (3) influencing and supporting other peoples, and (4) constructively resolving problems and conflicts in ways that bring people closer together and help the growth and development of the relationship (Johnson and Johnson 1975: 290).

From this definition, one could say that group practice with grieving and dying persons could truly be a growth experience. As the group counselor encourages the client to grow and move in and fill up the space between himself and the unknown, the client learns about his meaning and worth and increases his confidence in self and others.

It is the combination of trust and faith (Yalom 1975: 240) in self, others, and leader that encourages a person to explore and learn more of life and relationships.

Restitution

Restitution is assisted by the traditional preparation of religious practices, by the wake and funeral, and by condolences of friends. Caplan (as cited in Ren Kneisl 1976: 39) suggests another helpful way to allow the successful completion of anticipatory grief and postmortem grief would be "if the bereaved person were freed for a period from the demands of his job so that he could devote his energies to his 'grief work.'" This would permit the total input of "self" into the mourning response to loss and give time to aid adjustment to life. Restoration groups could possibly be sponsored at funeral homes and led by therapists and counselors in order to promote a healthy response to death. Anticipatory guidance could aid in adjusting to the impact of loss and help initiate the problem-solving process of preparation for personal or family member's death.

Parents, Children, and Adolescents, and Guilt

Knudson et al. state that mothers may have sought to gain renewed self-esteem through sharing experiences and feelings with another woman in a similar position. Perhaps knowing that someone else was encountering the same kind of crisis tended to make her feel less defeated and less vulnerable to negative feelings (as cited in Galiadi and Shandor 1969: 94).

This supports the need for a get-together time with parents and even with the adolescents and children themselves. Based upon the results of decreased psychic tension, the Oncology unit at the Hospital for Sick Children in Toronto has weekly parents group meetings and daily parent (child) team conferences about current complaints and emotional, physical, and cognitive states. Questions are honestly answered.

Adolescents and young adults are just coming into life—becoming productive, responsible persons capable of loving and procreation, of nurturing and developing their potentials. These clients may need more group and individual counseling, intervention, and activity to resolve the intensified feelings and fears of death.

Reasonably sensitive persons know well and feel deeply the pain and sorrow their death will cause. They feel guilty and responsible even when they know logically they are not....Always before there was a way out of guilt, an apology or explanation, a promise not to fail again, an act of special kindness in reparation....There is no other way to still feelings of guilt for going, for copping out of life, for becoming an emotional and financial burden and for that feeling of horrible helplessness inside (Kavanaugh 1974: 41).

Permission to Die

According to Kavanaugh (1974: 41): "Permission to die need never be spoken about or written....Permission to die is granted in all open and honest confrontations when patient and visitors accept the reality of needs of each other as together they willingly face the situation as it is."

Therapists can encourage small group permission activities—giving and receiving—by encouraging dyads and family groups to meet together privately and to discuss the patient's concerns and the family's remembrances and worries about the patient.

Once the permission to die is clearly granted, the dying patient can tackle the second major task, his personal work in voluntarily letting go. He begins with the outer circle of important acquaintances and business associates, now rarely seen, extending to close friends and family.

If there is to be a tranquility near death, all the dying can retain are what they truly own: their minds and loves, their memories and freedom and their faith (Kavanaugh 1974: 41).

It is the group leader's role to facilitate the strengthening of these personal entities in the patient and the remembrances of this free spirit by the family. Therapists may find that patients are despairing one minute and euphoric at others. The process of letting go is painful, and often most painful are the release of things like a favorite skateboard, baseball cards, favorite fishing lures or medals.

Denied the painful yet releasing and peaceful activities of "sharing all that I have," many clients carry on with jealousy, resentment, bitterness, and hoarding of life's treasures as disappointing substitutes far outreach the peace. The therapy group leader may not be able to do much with these people until it is too late.

Evaluation

The effectiveness of a therapeutic group is of interest to the leader, clients, and administrative sponsor.

Rewards of group participation are personal and individualized. Yalom states:

Members are satisfied with their groups (attracted to their groups and prone to continue membership in their groups) if:
1) They view the group as meeting their personal needs (i.e., their goals in therapy).
2) They derive satisfaction from their relationships with the other members.
3) They derive satisfaction from their participation in the group task.
4) They derive satisfaction from group membership vis-à-vis the outside world. Each of these factors, if absent or of negative valence, may outweigh the positive valence of the others and result in group termination (Yalom 1975: 239).

Feelings of satisfaction may not be totally positive on the part of the dying member if the outside world does not regard this group as highly valued or prestigious (Yalom 1975: 242). Shame and lack of support or outright dissonance from outsiders, who may mean well but fail to understand the work of the dying, inhibit the success of group activity for the members. A leader must, therefore, educate the public to the objectives, tasks, and aims of this special group and assess the group progress and cohesion.

Termination of group membership for the dying patient may be due to:

a) unsuccessful affiliation,
b) deterioration in physical, cognitive, or communication capabilities,
c) conflicts in levels of readiness to disclose, share, grow, confront,
d) lack of support and/or sabotage,
e) maladaptive communications and behaviors,
f) death.

In the group, termination might be best left to the readiness of the client. Yalom points out: "It is important that the therapist not bury the group too early, otherwise the group is in for several ineffective 'lame duck' sessions. One must find a way to hold the issue of termination before the group and yet help it keep working until the very last minute" (1975: 374). Sometimes it is in the very last minute that peacemaking and acceptance of death are achieved and families are calm and value the final rest of a loved one.

Group Activities
Group activities for the dying person, family members, and staff can begin with self-reflection upon personal qualities, fears, values, life-styles, accomplishments, and priorities.

Story telling, remembrances, and picture-emotive projection exercises can help to relate those areas of feelings associated with life, death, and meanings of "being." Unresolved crises or quiet people can be brought to consciousness by these activities.

In Epstein (1975), Simon (1974), and Stevens (1976), many strategies, obituary exercises, role-playing activities, scoring for observations, simulations, games, personal quizzes, discussion topics, creativity outlets, a repertoire of feeling responses, and intervention skills are clearly sequenced to facilitate growth and help.

Also of value are films, tape recordings, picture making, poetry writing, and diary notations. Through the activities together it is hoped that clients will move from "unbelief in self to happiness and belonging" (Maltz 1970).

References and Bibliography

Banet, A. G. 1974. "Therapeutic Interventions and the Perception of Process." *1974 Annual Handbook for Group Facilitators*. University Associates Publishing Inc., pp. 179-88.

Beachy, W. N. 1967. "Assisting the Family in Time of Grief." *Journal of The American Medical Association* (November), pp. 223-24.

Bliss, V. J. 1976. "Sharing Another's Death." *Nursing '76* (April) p. 30.

Brill, N. I. 1973. *Working with People, The Helping Process*. Philadelphia: Lippincott.

Curran, C. 1973. *Counseling-Learning, A Whole-Person Model for Education*. New York: Grune and Stratton.

Death and Dying Probe. 1974. *Nursing '74* (November) pp. 58-62.

Drummond, E. E. 1970. "Communication and Comfort for the Dying Patient." *Nursing Clinics of North America* 5 (1): 55-63.

Elfert, H. 1975. "The Nurse and the Grieving Parent." *The Canadian Nurse*. (February) p. 3031.

Epstein, C. 1975. *Nursing the Dying Patient*. Reston, Md.: Reston Publishing Company.

Feifel, H. 1977. *New Meanings of Death*. New York: McGraw-Hill.

Galiardi, D. and M. M. Shandor. 1969. "Interactions Between Two Mothers of Children Suffering from Incurable Cancer." *Nursing Clinics of North America*. 4 (1): 89-100.

Gray, V. R. 1974. "Grief." *Nursing '74*. (January) pp. 25-27.

Johnson, D. W. and F. P. Johnson. 1975. *Joining Together*. Englewood Cliffs, N. J.: Prentice-Hall.

Kavanaugh, R. E. 1976. "Dealing Naturally with the Dying." *Nursing '76*. (October) pp. 23-29.

Kavanaugh, R. E. 1974. "Facing Death." *Nursing '74*, (May) pp. 35-42.

Koop, C. E. 1969. "The Seriously Ill or Dying Child: Supporting the Patient and the Family. *Pedatric Clinics of North America*. 16 (3): 554-64.

Kopp, S. B. 1975. "The Refusal to Mourn," Unpublished dissertation summary from Cancer Clinic Metropolitan General Hospital, Windsor, Ontario.

Kübler-Ross, E. 1971. "Dying with Dignity." *The Canadian Nurse*. (October) pp. 31-35.

Maltz, M. 1970. *Psychocybernetics and Self Fulfillment*. New York: Grosset and Dunlop.

McElroy, C. 1975. "Caring for the Untreated Infant." *The Canadian Nurse*. (December) pp. 26-30.

Northrup, F. C. 1974. "The Dying Child." *American Journal of Nursing*. (June) pp. 1066-68.

Parkes, C. M. 1975. quoted in Feifel (p. 170).

Patterson, K. and M. Pomeroy. 1974. "S.I.D.S." *Nursing '74*. (May) pp. 85-88.

Pincus, L. 1976. *Death and the Family*. New York: Vintage Books.

Pinkel, D. 1976. "Treatment of Acute Leukemia." *Pediatric Clinics of North America* (February) pp. 117-30.

Pomeroy, M. 1969. "Sudden Death Syndrome." *American Journal of Nursing*. (September) pp. 1886-90.

Ren Kneisl, C. 1976. "Dying Patients and Their Families: How Staff Can Give Support." *Hospital Topics*. (November) pp. 37-39.

Rinear, E. 1975. "Helping the Survivors of Expected Death." *Nursing '75*. (March) pp. 60-65.

Rogers, J. and M. L. S. Vachon. 1975. "Nurses Can Help the Bereaved." *The Canadian Nurse*. (June) pp. 16-19.

Satir, V. 1967. *Conjoint Family Therapy*. Palo Alto, California: Science and Behavior Books.

Schmidt, J. "Availability: A Concept of Nursing Practice." *American Journal of Nursing*. (June) pp. 1087-89.

Schowalter, J. E. 1974. "Children's Reactions to Terminal Illness." *Pediatric Annals*. (November) pp. 93-101.

Simon, S. 1974. *Meeting Yourself Halfway*. Niles, Illinois: Argus Communications.

Stevens, J. 1976. *Awareness: Exploring, Experimenting, Experiencing*. New York: Bantam.

Waechter, E. 1971. "Children's Awareness of Fatal Illness." *American Journal of Nursing*. (June) pp. 1168-72.

Wiener, J. M. 1974. "Children and Dying." *Pediatric Annals* (November) pp. 83-92.

Williams, J. C. 1976. "Feelings of the Dying." *Nursing '76*. (March) pp. 52-56.

Yalom, I. D. 1975. *The Theory and Practice of Group Psychotherapy*. New York: Basic Books.

20

The Senior Citizen as a Hospice Volunteer

Audrey G. Harris

The purpose of this paper is to explore the feasibility of using the elderly as a resource for recruitment and training to become volunteer workers in the hospice concept of delivering health care and to identify the following: the characteristics of a volunteer, how a hospice program of care needs and uses the volunteer worker, the unique characteristics of the elderly in the role of volunteer, and the role the elderly can play as volunteer workers in the provision of hospice care.

Introduction

Since the turn of the century, individuals and groups of individuals have been donating their time and skills to help alleviate suffering and pain. The foci of their attention have broadened as the needs have been perceived. Beginning with shelters to aid the homeless, penniless alcoholic, volunteer groups have focused their efforts on fresh air camps, orphanages, working girls' homes, day nurseries, and hospitals. Volunteers are men and women, rich and poor, who have come from all kinds of backgrounds. They are not unique to any one educational level, socioeconomic stratum, race, religion, or age group.

In a health delivery setting, volunteers move to lend extra hands to aid the trained caregiver bring comfort and relief to the patient. They bring not only skills but also enthusiasm that says to the patient, "I care. I care enough to spend my time and energy, to do my best to help." Volunteers in health delivery systems can generally be described as individuals who are humanistic, altruistic, able to set aside time for service for others, mature, calm, and concerned. Many volunteers were previously employed in the health care system and continue to donate their skills and talents after retirement. Frequently, individuals volunteer as a result of experiences with relatives or friends who have been hospitalized or who have had long-term confinements in medical facilities. These individuals now ask, "What can I do? How can I help?" There are probably as many reasons for becoming a volunteer as there are opportunities to function as volunteers.

In a hospital or nursing home setting supervised volunteers perform a variety of tasks. They may run errands, read or talk with patients, help with the food tray, or perhaps make an empty bed. They may be asked to assist in transporting a patient to another part of the facility. While it is known that a large number of volunteers in hospitals and other medical facilities come from the aged population, it is difficult to cite numbers because few studies have been done related to the age of the volunteer. Other programs can be cited that seek only senior citizens as volunteer workers.

Foster Grandparent Program

The Foster Grandparent Program, a federally sponsored program under ACTION (an organization that unites all the federal volunteer agencies into one single effort devoted to making life better for people the world over), provides opportunities for senior citizens to help children in institutional settings. The role of the foster grandparent is to establish a one-to-one relationship with a child. The relationship is nurtured by love and understanding, by kindness, patience, and individual attention. Many children respond with genuine love for their foster grandparent. The relationship is developed by reading, talking, listening, taking walks together, playing games—anything that helps deepen the relationship. The federal guidelines for this program stipulate that the foster grandparent must be over 60 years of age.

Retired Senior Volunteer Program (RSVP)

The Retired Senior Volunteer Program is ACTION-funded and provides opportunities for older persons (over 60 years of age) to serve their communities. RSVP volunteers work in hospitals, schools, homes for the aged, foster homes, child care centers, libraries, museums, headstart programs, nutritional sites, and other agencies expressing need.

Senior Companions

The Senior Companion Program is a sister program to the Foster Grandparent Program. It is also funded by ACTION, and the volunteer must be at least 60 years of age. Here volunteers, as companions to the elderly, use their skills in a variety of ways to help the individual maintain independence.

Group Work with Older People Using Peer Counselors

The Continuum Center of Oakland University in Rochester, Michigan, has developed a model project of group counseling programs that train older men and women as peer counselors to bring mental health services to older people (Reiter and White 1978).

The overall experiences of these programs have been very positive.

A two-year study of the Foster Grandparent Program conducted in Detroit indicated that this program was having a major therapeutic effect on the social and emotional development of young institutionalized children who initially evidenced severe adjustment problems (Saltz 1968). The study further suggested that foster grandparents may have far-reaching beneficial effects on the age development of institutionalized children that assist them in coping with new experiences and environmental situations after the foster grandparent care is terminated.

Hospice Programs and Volunteers

The National Hospice Organization (NHO), incorporated in 1978, defines a hospice program as a centrally administered program of palliative and supportive services that provide physical, psychological, social, and spiritual care for dying persons and their families. Services are provided by a medically supervised interdisciplinary team of professionals and volunteers and are available in both the home and an inpatient setting. Home care is provided on a part-time, intermittent, regularly scheduled, and around-the-clock on-call basis. Bereavement services are also available to the family. Admission to hospice care is on the basis of patient and family needs.

The NHO hospice philosophy states that hospice affirms life and exists to provide support and care for persons in the last phases of incurable disease. Hospice recognizes dying as a normal process whether or not it results from disease. It neither hastens nor postpones death but has the hope and belief that through appropriate care and the promotion of a caring community sensitive to their needs patients and families may be free to attain a degree of mental and spiritual preparation for death that is satisfactory to them. Many different combinations of medical and support services are provided by hospices in a variety of settings. Medical services include home health care, skilled nursing care, aide care, home visits by physicians, psychiatric consultations, pain control, surgery, and radiation in those rare cases when it is necessary to relieve pain, physical therapy, occupational therapy, and inpatient and ambulatory services. Supportive services include bereavement followup, day care for patients, homemaker services, meal preparation at home, respite care for family members, and death education.

American hospice programs generally fall into the following five models:

–freestanding autonomous hospices
–freestanding hospices with hospital affiliation
–hospice unit within a hospital
–hospice teams within a hospital
–home care only

The General Accounting Office in its 1979 report to the Congress found hospices located in freestanding facilities, hospitals, skilled nursing facilities, health maintenance organizations, and home care agencies. Volunteers played a role in all of these various settings. In fact, the volunteer worker was an essential part of the interdisciplinary team, and the effective operation of a hospice program of care would be difficult without volunteer help as a result of costs incurred if they were to be replaced by paid personnel.

The National Hospice Organization in its 6th Revision of Standards and Criteria in February 1979 includes the volunteer in its interpretation of Standard No. 5: "Hospice care consists of a blending of professional and nonprofessional services." The interpretation of the standard describes the "core team" as consisting of ". . . the patient and the patient's family, the attending physician, nurse, social worker, patient care coordinator, volunteer director and clergy. The significance of each of these professional resources will be considered equal in the functioning of the Hospice team. The team (including volunteers) will work as an interdisciplinary unit with a common commitment to the care of the patient and family. . . . "

The interpretation of Standard No. 5 goes on to say:

The volunteers are to be carefully selected, trained, and supervised by a member of the core team, the Director of Volunteers. The volunteer staff may consist of professionals and nonprofessionals. It will complement and support the paid professional and nonprofessional staff. The volunteer staff will participate in continuing education programs designed to enhance their effectiveness as part of the Hospice patient care team. These programs are designed to improve and develop specific skills and sensitivities in such areas as individual and group dynamics, supportive counseling, and listening skills.

The volunteer staff provide services under the direction of the Patient Care Coordinator and the Director of Volunteers. The volunteers attend regular supervisory and patient care conferences. They will also contribute to the patient record documenting Hospice intervention.

There are a variety of helping services that the volunteer can provide to the patient and family, the professional team members, and to the hospice unit itself. Not all of the volunteer's work is concerned with direct patient contact. This is extremely important to keep in mind for those individuals who want to volunteer their time and efforts but do not feel comfortable working with patients. The range of tasks may encompass shopping, typing, driving, baby-sitting, pet-sitting, telephoning, filing, or any number of day-to-day chores necessary in running a household or office.

Hospice volunteers, both lay and professional, are traditionally recruited from various sources. Family members and friends of patients and former patients represent a large portion of volunteers. Invitations offered to volunteer groups or individuals who regularly serve in hospitals and nursing home settings have yielded a sizable number. The Connecticut Hospice, Inc. (Cox 1979) reports that volunteers also apply as a result of media presentations describing the hospice and its program. There is usually a wide range of backgrounds, nationalities, and ages among the hospice volunteer workers, but the source that does *not* appear to have been considered is the elderly.

The hospice program of care has been offered as a more cost-effective alternative to the care generally provided in the acute-care setting. Although the GAO study indicated that it was difficult to compare these costs, it did find that the operating costs were in direct relation to the ratio of paid to volunteer staff.

Table 20.1 gives statistics on these staffs as reported in the General Accounting Office study. Another study (Holden 1976) suggests that the volunteer-to-professional staff ratio in most hospices is approximately 12 to 1. In any event, it can readily be seen how the use of volunteers can foster the cost effectiveness of the program.

Those programs that deliberately sought and used the elderly as volunteers have demonstrated the unique effectiveness of the aged. We

Table 20.1 Number and Percent of Paid and Volunteer Staff by Major Occupational in 53 Hospices

	Paid Workers		Volunteers	
Occupational group	Number	Percent	Number	Percent
Physicians	13.0	4	138	6
Nursing/aide staff	181.5	53	305	14
Therapists/technicians	6.2	2	27	1
Social/psychlogical staff	19.2	6	208	9
Personal care/administrative/ clerical staff	120.8	35	1,575	70
Total	340.7	100	2,251	100

have seen the elderly interact successfully with different age segments of society, and we should now consider the suitability of using this population in caring for the dying patient. After all, terminal illness occurs within all age segments of the population.

In assessing the health care needs of the inner city residents, the City of Detroit Health Department recognized its high population of extreme age groups—the aged and the young. Detroit is an economically depressed area with underemployed and/or near-poverty-level citizens composing a majority of its population. Characteristics of these population groupings usually include a high proportion of recipients of public assistance, including Old Age Assistance and Aid to Dependent Children. The level of health care is characteristically low with an expected high morbidity and mortality rate. The cancer mortality rate, for example, is 301.7 per 100,000.

Frequently, it has been found that the economic status of this near-poverty and poverty-level population has created and encouraged a close-knit family support network that is an essential element in the patient socialization process. Minority extended families often consist of two to three generations living in the same household. Removal from this socialization pattern into the isolated impersonal medical care facility increases anxiety and alienation for the patient and often cuts children and/or grandchildren in the same family and household adrift.

In its commitment to the hospice concept of care for the terminally ill patient, the Detroit health department sought methods that would deliver this kind of care and preserve the positive benefits from the multigenerational interaction. In July 1978, the Detroit health department formed a coalition of public and private sectors consisting of the health department, Wayne State University, Comprehensive Health Planning Council of Southeastern Michigan, and the Neighborhood Services Organization. This group endeavored to develop a day care center to provide services to 15 terminally ill adult patients and their families and 30 children. The coalition felt that the integration of children into what is primarily an aged population would allow both age groups to give and receive emotional support from each other.

Even though the Detroit example places the aged in the position of patient, it is mentioned to point out the value of recognizing and using the mature, empathetic, and often intuitive skills of the elderly.

Summary

The hospice program of care relies heavily on the volunteer worker for the effective delivery of services to the terminally ill patient and family. The mature, empathetic, caring senior citizen has demonstrated a willingness and capability of serving as a volunteer worker in a variety of settings and with a variety of age groups. It would seem worthwhile that further exploration be made to assess the use of the elderly as volunteers in the provision of a hospice program of care.

References

Cox, M. S. 1979. "The Connecticut Hospice, Inc. Volunteer Program." New Haven: Hospice Institute for Education, Training and Research, Inc.

"Day Care Center for Terminally Ill Persons and Children in a Specific Geographic Area of the City of Detroit." 1978. Health Finances Research Demonstration and Experiments of the Health Care Financing Administration, DHEW.

Holden, C. 1976. "Hospices: For the Dying, Relief from Pain and Fear." *Science* (July).

Reiter, S. and B. White, 1978. Paper presented at the 26th Annual Conference of the National Council on Aging. St. Louis, Missouri (April).

Saltz, R. 1968. "Foster Grandparents and Institutionalized Young Children: Two Years of a Foster Grandparent Program." Detroit, Michigan: Merrill-Palmer Institute (September).

Bibliography

Newell, M. M., H. H. Naylor, B. Marcus, A. H. Kutscher, D. J. Cherico, and I. B. Seeland, eds. 1980. *The Role of the Volunteer in the Care of the Terminal Patient and the Family*. New York: Arno Press.

Part V

Patients and Illnesses

21

Helping Preterminal and Terminal Cancer Patients Function Within the Community

Martin Blackstein and Eleanor Wasserman

As a medical oncologist and nurse coordinator we have examined more than six years of patient care involving more than 500 terminally ill cancer patients. The emphasis of the care has been to keep patients functioning within the community for as long as possible. This review served as the background for the discussion that follows. We focus here on the time interval between the patient's diagnosis and his death.

The needs of the individual patient and family were assessed by a nurse based in an ambulatory oncology unit; use of community resources enabled the preterminal and terminal phases of the disease to be experienced at home. The oncology service is based in and run through the facilities of the Mount Sinai Hospital (Toronto), a 510-bed general hospital within the University of Toronto Teaching Hospitals system. Several years ago an oncology division (jointly sponsored by the departments of medicine and surgery of this hospital) was founded. The unit is currently housed in its outpatient department and records more than

3,000 patient visits per annum. Within the University of Toronto and numerous outside agencies, the oncology division actively participates in the support of recognized clinical trials in cancer chemotherapy. Our major concerns have also been to provide a high standard of care in terms of actual treatment and to assist the patient and family in maintaining a good quality of life.

The oncology service at Mount Sinai is somewhat unique. Owing to the commitment of the physicians, most patients are followed by a single physician until the time of death even though active treatment may be discontinued months before. A majority of patients who have been referred to the unit continue to be seen there and get medical and support services from individuals within the unit. One of our concerns has been whether the quality of a patient's life is more meaningful when care is provided from a community base and at home as opposed to an alternative base providing institutional palliative terminal care.

The medical oncologist has at all times attempted to actively involve the patient in decisions concerning further treatment in the form of chemotherapy, radiotherapy, or surgery. In addition, the option of home care and continuing ambulatory (outpatient) support, with the option of hospitalization at Mount Sinai for a very limited (less than three weeks) terminal stay or placement in an appropriate chronic care facility much earlier in the course of the illness, is given to the patient. Over the last six years we have emphasized the option of developing support systems within the community. The ideal patient for this program is usually one under the age of sixty with strong family support who has been informed of his diagnosis and has accepted the further treatment programs offered. In addition, the support of a concerned family physician who is kept informed about treatment schedules and complications is of considerable importance.

We believe, however, that it is the program that enables the patient and his family to remain together in the community; a major component of this program involves an early meeting between the patient, family, and nurse coordinator. The first meeting often takes place at the most stressful time of first diagnosis, and meetings continue on an irregular basis in anticipation of further crises (such as failure of the existing treatment protocol) and finally because of lack of further efficacious treatment.

The nurse coordinator is available at all times to work as an advocate for both the patient and the family within the complex system. This is particularly important to cancer patients, many of whom feel that they have lost control of their fate. The coordinator knows her patient population very well early in the course of the illness and tries to assess problems before they develop into a crisis. Individually, both the physician and nurse coordinator meet with the patient and/or family after the patient has been informed of his diagnosis, prognosis, and treatment plan; and the coordinator keeps constant contact with the physician. This initial re-review, although difficult and time-consuming for the staff, is critical. The majority of patients, no matter how intelligent or knowledgeable, are unable because of the stress to absorb more than a fraction of the information conveyed to them in the early stages of their illness.

Many patients consider their coordinator the link to the physician and the hospital system. They feel comfortable staying in the community as long as this relationship can be maintained. Although preparatory counseling sessions to assist families, to help patients at difficult times in the illness, and to prepare the family for the eventual outcome are held on an irregular basis, they are, however, planned beforehand— often on consultation with a community-based (home care) nurse who has been involved in the home and may be aware of problems not apparent to the hospital-based staff. Bereavement followup is also done by the treatment team (usually the nurse coordinator alone) and shows significant results because of family familiarity with our personnel. We are thus capable of intervening at another critical point to prevent problems of unresolved grief.

This system has proved to be an effective model for a university general hospital. While supporting the patient and family through the final illness, it stresses family involvement during all phases of the illness. The responses from patients and families indicate appreciation for the definitive care given and the process of easing the concerns of all involved.

22

Caring for the Patient With Pulmonary Emphysema

Hylan A. Bickerman

Pulmonary emphysema is a relative newcomer to the list of chronic, life-threatening diseases of man. In the decade following World War II, it became more fashionable to group a number of pulmonary disorders characterized by obstruction or limitation in airflow under the general term of chronic obstructive pulmonary disease (COPD). It has become increasingly evident that emphysema and chronic bronchitis, representing the major disorders in COPD, are rapidly growing adult health problems not only in the more industrialized nations of the world but also in the undeveloped countries. Even though estimates of the total public health problem in the United States are incomplete, all data indicate that perhaps four to six million individuals have well-established disease, and approximately two to three times this number have early or latent disease. The preclinical course of most patients who develop severe, disabling COPD may be quite variable. Some show a steady decline in lung function throughout their adult life, others may retain normal function and then deteriorate rapidly just prior to onset of clinical symptoms, while others may have episodic attacks of broncho-constriction for many years before chronic, irreversible disease takes place.

On epidemiologic grounds, there is strong evidence for an increase in incidence and mortality of emphysema. It is now estimated that 10 to 20 percent of the urban male population over the age of 50 has some degree of emphysema, and the New York City health department reported a tenfold increase in mortality during the 1960s. COPD is now second only to the cardiovascular diseases (including stroke) as a cause of total disability under Social Security.

This prelude to the care of the preterminally and terminally ill patient is intended to emphasize that by the time the patient, who is generally in his late fifties or early sixties, first presents himself to the physician with chronic progressive shortness of breath and a troublesome cough, he has lost approximately 60 to 70 percent of his normal pulmonary function over a 20- to 30-year period. At this point, he is usually severely disabled, anxious, and depressed about the progressive nature of his downhill course. This is compounded by the pessimistic attitude of many physicians who, having told the patient he has pulmonary emphysema, intimate that little can be done for him. It is little wonder that such patients have equated their disease with end-stage cancer.

While the prognosis for the patient with advanced disease is poor, with a 41 percent survival at the end of 5 years, and only 17 percent at the end of 10 years (Sahn et al. 1980), as compared with healthy individuals in the same age group whose survival rates were 86 and 69 percent, respectively, the physician is faced with providing the best health care possible for these individuals so that they may experience a reasonable quality of life in their remaining years.

In an Aspen Lung Conference on COPD, the various risk factors for the initiation and progression of COPD were discussed (Woolcock 1980). These factors, including cigarette smoking, infection, genetic trait, and occupational and environmental hazards, are responsible for the destruction of the lung morphology by elastase and other proteases. The defect in elastic recoil with disruption of alveoli is responsible for airflow limitation, increased work of breathing, abnormal gas exchange with hypoxemia and hypercapnea, and severe progressive dyspnea on the slightest exertion. The patient with advanced COPD becomes a bedridden respiratory cripple who requires the full use of the accessory muscles of respiration in order to maintain adequate ventilation.

Grant and his co-workers (1980) suggest that, in addition to its cardiopulmonary effects, the hypoxia of advanced COPD results in neuropsychologic defects resembling organic brain dysfunction. The highest cognitive functions, reasoning and perceptual motor integration, are most seriously affected, while memory appears to be relatively spared. Many of these patients also experience substantial emotional disturbances that affect their quality of life, such as mood changes with depression and inflexibility; decreased social and family interrelationships; poor basic behavioral functioning, including self-care skills and mobility; and a diminished capacity to engage in hobbies and recreational activities. While this may result from hypoxia of the limbic system and other portions of the brain that mediate emotional behavior, it is also apparent that many of the emotional changes may be secondary to the severe restriction on activity imposed by the disease itself. Frustration, irritability, and depression would be common in such a setting.

In 1974, I was asked to draw up a proposal for a special care, or demonstration unit, at the Francis Delafield Hospital as part of a cardiopulmonary center to be established at the Columbia-Presbyterian Medical Center and affiliated hospitals. The aim of this unit was to employ techniques of comprehensive respiratory care to the long-term management of chronic respiratory insufficiency due to COPD, in agreement with the following statement of the Committee on Pulmonary Rehabilitation of the American College of Chest Physicians:

Pulmonary rehabilitation may be defined as an art of medical practice wherein an individually tailored, multi-disciplinary program is formulated which through accurate diagnosis, therapy, emotional support, and education, stabilizes or reverses both the physio- and psychopathology of advanced pulmonary disease and attempts to return the patient to the highest possible functional capacity allowed by his pulmonary handicap and overall life situation (Petty 1977).

The objectives to be tested in this unit were:

1. Evaluation of various techniques employed in the management program with respect to (a) immediate and long-term benefit, (b) ease of performance, (c) degree of cooperation required, (d) need for training and time required; and (e) cost.

2. Can the quality of life be improved by (a) increase in exercise

tolerance, (b) acquisition of hobbies, (c) overcoming depression, (d) improving family and social relationships, and (e) returning to part-time sedentary work?

3. Can the clinical course be stabilized so that following discharge, patients can be managed in their home environment with a suitable home care program and thus avoid frequent admission to the hospital?

To be eligible for admission to the unit, patients must have a documented history of COPD and be recovering from or be in borderline respiratory failure. The modalities of care to be employed include:

a) measures to lower airways resistance by pharmacologic agents, including therapeutic aerosols;
b) facilitation of bronchial drainage by a variety of chest physiotherapy measures, as well as the use of humidifying and mucolytic agents;
c) low-flow oxygen therapy employing accurately calibrated delivery systems with frequent monitoring;
d) respiratory muscle rest through the use of various mechanical ventilators such as the tank respirator, body Cuirass, and pressure-limited IPPB devices;
e) tracheostomy care where indicated;
f) a graded exercise program with and without oxygen to improve general physical fitness (combined with measures designed to improve diaphragmatic mobility and breathing retraining);
g) education, including psychological, social, and occupational counseling.

The unit was to be organized so as to provide for a minimum of six beds with additional space for a central nurses station and staff personnel, as well as a supporting laboratory. The arrangement of beds could be two double and two single rooms or six individual rooms. The personnel for such a unit for 24-hour daily coverage would include a clinical chest physician as director, one fellow in pulmonary medicine, three staff physicians (one resident and two interns), one head nurse with special training or experience in respiratory care, four RN staff nurses, four LPNs or nurses aides, one chest physiotherapist, one respiratory therapist, and one pulmonary function technician. Social service, dietetic, psychiatric, and religious counseling, and occupational therapy services will be provided on a consultation basis to help with family and social interrelationships.

200   Hylan A. Bickerman

While such a unit is designed to be intensive with respect to personnel rather than technology, the patient with severe pulmonary insufficiency requires many aids to breathing, such as oxygen therapy and mechanical devices, to achieve a reasonable degree of comfort.

The goals of such a unit would be to provide a special care type of facility for the management of the patient with severe COPD that could be coordinated with a number of clinical research projects designed to evaluate the cost effectiveness of various treatment modalities, new devices, and pharmacologic agents; and to determine the minimum amount of respiratory support needed to maintain the patient in a home care program before discharge. It is hoped that such a facility would make it possible to return these patients to their homes and maintain them in their familiar community environment with backup from the unit's home care service so that frequent hospitalizations are avoided and there is a minimal disruption of the family unit. In special instances, patients who are discharged to their homes could return several nights per week for respiratory rest in the tank respirator.

There have been a number of pilot projects designed to provide specialized care for advanced COPD in both the hospital setting and home care service (Petty et al. 1969; Report of Intersociety Commission 1974). Most of these were short term because of expiration of grants from the U. S. Public Health Service. However, there were positive trends indicating that survival time could be prolonged with improvement in the quality of life, and the number of hospitalizations and days hospitalized were significantly reduced.

References

Grant, I., R. K. Heaton, A. J. McSweeney, K. M. Adams, and R. M. Timms. 1980. "Brain Dysfunction in COPD." *Chest* (Feb.) 77:308, Suppl.

Petty, T. L. 1977. "Pulmonary Rehabilitation." *Respiratory Care* 22 (1):68.

Petty, T. L., L. M. Nett, M. M. Finigan, G. A. Brink, and P. R. Corsello. 1969. "A Comprehensive Care Program for Chronic Airway Obstruction." *Annals of Internal Medicine* (June) 70:1109.

Report of Intersociety Commission for Heart Disease Resources. 1974. "Community

Resources for Rehabilitation of Patients with Chronic Obstructive Pulmonary Diseases and Cor Pulmonale." *Circulation* 49:A-1.

Sahn, S. A., L. M. Nett, and T. L. Petty. 1980. "Ten Year Followup of a Comprehensive Rehabilitation Program for Severe COPD."*Chest* (Feb.) 778:311S-314S, Suppl.

Woolcock, A. J. 1980. Conference Summary—22nd Aspen Lung Conference. *Chest* (Feb.) 77:326, Suppl.

23

Illness Factors in ALS—
A Neuromuscular Disease

Joan E. Anderson

Understandably, the biological processes involved with, and the nature
and course related to, a specific disease are important factors in the
planning of a medical program related to that particular disease. Almost
without exception, each type of medical disorder requires its own unique
protocol of medical intervention consisting of such variables as drug
therapy, nursing care, surgical techniques, and rehabilitation. As a
matter of course, large-scale medical facilities take these factors into
consideration as they set up various wards and specialized units. However, often absent in this planning are both a consideration of the social
dimensions of disease in general and any specific disease in particular.
The following paper, offered as one approach toward a redress of this
situation, is an examination of the social or "illness" aspects of one
neuromuscular disease—amyotrophic lateral sclerosis (ALS), a fatal,
progressively deteriorating disorder.

Historically, the exclusion of social factors occurred when the
medical profession abandoned its holistic analysis of disease processes
in favor of the single cause or specific etiological approach indicative of
the microbiotic era of research. Under this medical or engineering
approach to disease, the patient lost his social character as emphasis

shifted to biological attributes. For the most part, medical care and its delivery have also followed this particular approach.

But today it is the contention of many social scientists, health care personnel, as well as physicians, that systematic inattention to the social dimensions of disease, what I refer to in this paper as the "illness" correlates of disease, is in part responsible for noncompliance by patient and family to medical directives, dissatisfaction of consumers with medical services, and also frustration of physicians and staff. Furthermore, lack of an inclusion of social factors has also been cited as an impediment to the discovery of the etiology of many specific diseases.

Planning for the care and support of patients, especially those with a life-threatening disease, demands that we examine these illness factors. Illness, in very broad terms, is the way the sick person, his family, and his social network perceive, label, explain, evaluate, and respond to disease; in other words, it is the experience and the societal reaction to biological disorder or perceived disorder. Thus "disease" is used to indicate that one is referring to a concept that has originated and is contained mainly within the domain of the medical profession; "illness" indicates, on the other hand, that one is dealing with the domain of the patient and his experience of his "disease." It must be cautioned that in actuality they are not totally mutually exclusive, for neither disease nor illness is a thing, an entity; instead they are different social constructions of reality. (Kleinman 1978)

My approach to ALS as an illness developed out of my work with ALS patients at two metropolitan medical facilities—one specifically geared to research and the other to a combination of research and the psychosocial aspects of this disorder. Despite differences in their basic orientation, they both failed to deal with the patient and his experience of the disease. There was an observable inconsistency between the professional evaluation of ALS and that of the patient and his family. Ironically, these discrepancies were problematic not only for the patient and staff relationships but also for the two projects, as dissatisfaction impeded participation and medical followups necessary for the continuation of the projects.

One specific example from this investigation points to the need for an inclusion of the patient's experience of ALS. It was found that there were two aspects of the illness correlate that ran counter to expectation based on the clinical picture of ALS; in other words, there were two aspects that had no basis in the biological dysfunctions associated with this disorder. They are loss of memory and a decline in the ability by males to perform sexually. In a study undertaken by this author of 43 patients (25 males, 18 females), 10 (40 percent) of the males complained of a loss of sexual functioning; and 30 (69 percent) of all patients referred to having a loss of memory. Various hypotheses can be offered with regard to these results: loss of job, social position, familiar routine, responsibility, and/or the threat of further disability and eventual death. All 43 of these patients had lost little or no physical functioning at the time of their interview. The important point here is that these complaints were for the most part ignored because the therapeutic programs were directly related to the clinical picture of this disease.

The following brief encapsulation will set the stage for an analysis of ALS as an illness. For some still unexplained reason, ALS attacks motor neurons (the nerve cells controlling muscles) in the brain and spinal cord to produce progressive muscle weakness and wasting. Symptoms vary, depending on the site of initial involvement, but regardless of the primary location of degeneration, the motor neurons throughout the nervous system are involved before death. ALS causes its victims to slowly lose the use of their hands, arms, legs, power of speech, ability to swallow, and finally the ability to sustain life. During this time the patient's mind remains clear, the sensory apparatus intact. Death results from inanition, paralysis of the accessory muscles of respiration, or from aspiration pneumonia.

In terms of professional medical care and/or equipment, the average ALS patient may require all or part of the following aides:

rehabilitation
respiratory therapy
nutritional guidance
occupational therapy
communication facilitation
minor surgical procedures for aid in
    breathing and/or nutritional assimilation
round-the-clock nursing

Three distinctive features of ALS serve to differentiate the care needed by these patients from that which is involved with many other terminal diseases: first, there is little or no pain associated with this disorder; second, many of these patients suffer from an inability to communicate, either vocally or by gesture; and third, there is an extensive and progressive loss of physical mobility, often occurring early in the disease course. Other aspects, such as the lack of medical intervention to be able to slow the progression of the disease or to offer a hope for remission, add unique psychological dimensions. These aspects, as are discussed in this paper, present a series of specific illness manifestations that also require professional consideration.

With this brief medical description of ALS in mind, let us now examine ALS as an illness, that is, how the patient experiences his "disease." Whereas under the disease concept the defining characteristics of ALS in terms of initial symptoms are expressed in biological malfunctions of either the whole body (fatigue) or of its separate parts (weakness in hands, legs, or voice); the patient, on the other hand, is concerned with the manifestations of these dysfunctions in terms of losses in ability to work, play, and attend to the activities of everyday living and social activities. In a random sample of 44 (total 88) patient interviews in my study, the recording of initial symptoms fell into the following categories:

Change in Ability to:	Total: 44
perform job	19
travel to job	12
participate in sports	6
write, comb hair, dress children	7

While the breakdown may be of particular interest in determining the priorities of this particular patient population, the manner in which these symptoms were phrased is also important. For example:

I noticed I couldn't jog as far. I used to be able to go longer.
My tennis game was off.
I had difficulty cutting at work (patient was a leather cutter).

As the disease progresses, the patient relays his increase of symptoms in the same manner.

For the patient, loss of social functioning is progressive. It differs between patients in terms of rate, degree, and kind, depending on the situation (social and/or psychological) that existed prior to the illness. Each loss of physical functioning produces a concomitant loss for the patient in such things as the ability to feed, dress, or to care for one's person. An accumulation of any of these variables often results in the loss of a total social function. For example, the patient who no longer has control of his hands and has difficulty climbing stairs may be forced to leave his job, if that job requires fine motor coordination or the job access requires the patient to climb many stairs. The physical space of the patient shrinks as he is no longer able to travel freely. Decline of social space accompanies this loss as the patient is not able to continue many of his former social relationships. Since the majority of ALS patients are males within the work force, an accumulation of small losses or one major loss results in a forced retirement from the work force.

The following is a portion of a transcript from a patient's examination at a major research facility. The patient, a male aged 53, was a jewelry designer until problems with fine motor coordination forced him to retire. The time elapsed during this examination was 2 1/2 hours, approximately 30 minutes of which was directly concerned with medical evaluation, the rest with the patient's loss of certain social functions.

Dr.:   Well, M, how are things going?

Pat.:   Well, I still feel the same. I can't find anything different. You said I should come in for a few days for a urine test.

Dr.:   No, not a urine test, but I would like you to come in for a couple of days.

Wife: His problem is with his time. He doesn't have anything to do. All he does is go shopping. He takes $20 and goes to the shopping center. I never see what he buys, but he comes home with one cent. He has nothing to do all day.

Pat.:   You work for so many years and finally get to retire—it is something you have dreamt about—having all that free time—but it is too much. There is just so much you can do at home, so many books you can read or projects you can do. There is just too much time. And anyway, I wasn't ready to retire, I planned it to happen much later.

Wife: If he had something to do, he wouldn't worry so much.

Pat.:   (now noticeably upset—shifts body forward and raises voice) I worked all my life, 50 years, now do you want me to go out and work again? What do you want me to do—go around and collect for MDA? Go around with a cup to the bowling alley and collect money?

Wife: You're only 53 years old, you weren't out in the street working for 50 years.

Pat.:   (again raising his voice) Why does she want me to work, I can't work. It's her job, that's the problem: she has a full-time job and doesn't get home until 8. She wants to get away. How am I so aggravating? I greet her just like the dog...friendly. I'm a very friendly guy.

Wife: That's it, he is just waiting for me to cook and clean for him.

Dr.:   Are you saying he is too dependent?

Wife: Yes, you know, an Italian mother pours her husband his wine, he can't do it himself (points to her husband). He can't even pour water.

Pat.:   (at this point he moves up further in his chair, raises his hand and shakes it) I don't depend on you. I can do it myself.

Dr.:   Maybe you should get a job—how about opening a bookie joint.

Pat.:   (laughs) Better yet, they have this massage parlor near where we live, maybe I'll run that.

Dr.:   We don't really want you to get a job, we just want to keep your mind busy.

Wife: I tried to get him to go to work at the Mall near us where they sell kits to make your own jewelry, but he wouldn't. They give classes to teach you how to do it, and I thought that M could teach.

Pat.:   How could I (looks at hands and moves fingers)? I can't stand either, my legs won't hold up.

Dr.:   That's true, you couldn't do fine work, but there is no reason why you couldn't do selling. With your knowledge and experience, you would be a tremendous asset to any firm, especially with your outgoing personality.

Pat.:   But I can't stand for any amount of time.

Dr.:   But a lot of selling can be done while you're sitting down.

Pat.:   If I could do a lot of things myself, everything would be all right.

Dr.:   M, deep down you don't want to.

Pat.:   I should be the breadwinner. I don't want to be reminded that she is doing things; she makes it seem that she is doing things; she makes it seem that she is the only one doing something here. How can she be doing everything when she is out there all the time. She makes me feel that (gestures with hands) low.

From this brief conversation, it is not surprising to note that this patient experienced both a sexual loss and a loss of memory, both of which were expressed in all his examinations.

The most severe loss experienced by the ALS patient is loss of the ability to communicate. This usually occurs only prior to death, but with a bulbar form of ALS, verbal communication is the first loss, while the patient retains the use of his hands for manual communication. Loss of the ability to communicate one's thoughts and needs is the ultimate in alienation. The patient who is not able to express his needs leaves his ministrations to the total discretion of others. Since eye movement remains intact, some system can be used to signal discomfort. But for the most part, this type of system is limited to the immediate family, for most professionals involved with these patients are not familiar with the particular types of communication systems.

Depending on the situation of each particular patient, ALS as an illness can be viewed as a series of social losses, each of which has a distinct set of repercussions for both the patient and the family. For example, as the patient becomes progressively unable to care for himself, to perform the basic activities of daily living, there must be some compensation for these losses. In other words, someone must dress, feed, and attend to the patient's bodily functions. This can be seen as occurring on a continuum from help in minor areas, as doing buttons or zippers, to the total care required at the end stages, when the patient needs help to breathe and keep his air passages free from phlegm. For the family this decline requires tremendous expenditures of time, energy, commitment, as well as financial outlays; while for the patient, it spells a growing and constant dependency. In light of this, one of my initial findings—that these patients and their families presented an overwhelming concern not with impending death but with living until death—is most understandable.

In very broad terms, the illness aspects of ALS that require palliative measures, so to speak, are displacement, isolation, alienation, and dependency. These four factors must be considered as being mediated by the culture and society, as well as by the immediate environment within which the afflicted individual is found. In other words, illness seen as a state of social dysfunction is, in part, defined by the expectation of society and involves the state of relations with others, as well as by one's own self-expectations. These factors can, in fact, be generalized to all classes of illness. The leading social analysts of our time remind us that they are part of the social relationships engendered by a society and replicated within a medical system in which sickness is an occasion for both the isolation of the individual and for his or her subjection to medical "management." The specifics of a particular illness serve only to determine the form and degree of displacement, isolation, alienation, and dependency. ALS appears to be at the extreme negative end of this continuum.

Thus, we find that intervention directed toward an amelioration of these illness factors requires innovative programs able to go beyond the traditional medical and social service support. The key here is self-determination, for programs that consider ways of helping the patient remain in control of his or her physical and social environment can serve to decrease the negative stigma associated with dependency, as well as to alter the effects of loss of status, position, communication, and social contact.

At first glance, there appears to be a contradiction in this approach. How can the need for autonomy on the part of the patient be reconciled with his obvious, and in the case of the ALS patient, overwhelming need for support? I believe the contradiction is only superficially apparent, for the problem is not that society (and its subsystem, the medical system) generates dependency but that it generates a specific kind of dependency, one that has a negative social impact. Dependency is an intrinsic fact of social life; it is implicit within the category "social." We need now to envision a medical care system able to acknowledge our need for autonomous control over our own care and well-being, while at the same time, it accepts our need for dependency; one that enhances autonomy but that, when we do find the need to accept help, to be dependent, can deal with that need in a dignified and nurturing way. To truly meet the needs of the ALS patient, as well as all other patients with life-threatening illnesses, our proposed Continuing Care Service must consider providing an environment able to foster self-help and mutual help.

In the final analysis, the "how" of the delivery of services may well be as important, if not more important, than the content of these services. The following example illustrates one approach to the delivery of care within a relationship of self-help and mutual help. One of the major decisions to be made in the care of the ALS patient is whether to plan for the patient's final care and eventual death at home or within the hospital. Too often this planning is done for the patient and not with the patient.

For example, reflecting the latest concern for a "death at home," the largest ALS clinic in the metropolitan area offers this concept to all its patients as the best possible solution. The functioning of the clinic also operates toward this goal. This may well be the best possible solution for many patients but by no means for all. But more important is the fact that this is offered to the patient as a predetermined and evaluated solution as opposed to its being arrived at by a joint decision-making process. An alternative and more viable approach would be to extend to the patient and his family information on the alternatives of care available and to explore with them the ramifications of these possible decisions. Thus, for example, when the patient requires help and is placed in a dependent situation, he has defined that situation based on personal preference, not arbitrary assignment. This lessens the negative connotations involved.

By being denied the control over the manner in which he will live until death, the patient remains entrenched in the illness factors of displacement, isolation, alienation, and dependency. If any organized caregiving service is to meet its goal of achieving the highest level of patient care, then, at least for the ALS patient, the patient's input must be seen as an essential ingredient within the planning and execution of care.

Reference

Kleinman, A. 1978. "Concepts and a Model for the Comparison of Medical Systems." *Social Sciences and Medicine* 1(12):85-93.

Part VI

Alternatives to In-Hospice Care

24

Some Questions About Hospice Development

Donald Malafronte

As a hospital consultant, I have been involved in health planning for several hospice programs for hospitals and for long-term care institutions for the elderly. Is the interest in hospice warranted? Will the hospice movement grow, and will hospitals benefit from promoting it and participating in it? As a consultant, I must tell those seeking advice that there is as yet no truly definitive answer. The National Hospice Organization, the National Cancer Institute, and other agencies agree that a hospice is not so much a place as it is a concept of care. This has surprised many administrators.

Consultants, like myself, also remind inquirers that American Medical Association guidelines adopted in 1973 state that "the employment of extraordinary means to prolong the life of the body when there is irrefutable evidence that death is imminent is the decision of the patient and/or his immediate family." This suggests that the medical approach is not always the most appropriate and that hospitals may not be the best sponsors. This should be considered before there is a rush forward to establish hospices. The General Accounting Office has told Congress that the object of the care is to make the patient's remaining days as comfortable and meaningful as possible and to help the family cope with the stress involved. We consultants think in terms of what the people who have planned the hospice in New Haven say about hospice and the control of total pain—physical, emotional, social, spiritual, financial, and bureaucratic—all the pains that the terminal patient and his family must face and that must be faced as well by the would-be sponsors.

The wave of hospice interest among hospitals arises from a number of sources, including a desire to serve terminally ill patients better. However, it arises also from a desire to gain extra federal dollars or be in a position to do so by initiating or expanding home care services or filling empty beds. There is also the general desire to stay current, to avoid missing out on what may be limited by regulation in the future, or to gain a competitive advantage.

The following questions are of value in hospice development. *First*, have the medical and moral issues inherent in any hospice approach been considered? Hospice care is at odds with the normal hospital and medical care business of curing disease, repairing injury, and saving and extending life. A case can be made for finding other sponsors, as in the English experience.

Second, what is the hospital presently doing for its terminally ill patients? It does not take a federal grant to adopt a hospice concept, nor does it take one to install services based on the concept. Much of what constitutes hospice care can be provided without new sources of revenue within existing hospital systems. A hospital that wants to provide basic hospice care needs only to gain agreement among its own staff and board. No certificate of need is required to rethink, reorganize, and resystemize how a hospital treats the dying, their relatives, and their friends.

The *third* question is: Who is going to do the work? Is there a group at the hospital currently working with the terminally ill who are willing and able to do the committee and other work necessary to establish a hospice? Are any of them influential? In most cases, the work will fall to two or three nurses or two or three doctors, the social service department, the home care department (if there is one), and the assistant administrator. Can they be spared for the job? Do they have the time and the power to get it done?

Fourth, is the hospital prepared to carry the program beyond home care arrangements? It is likely that hospice programs in the United States will consist largely of home care. It appears to be the best and most practical way of proceeding. However, it is our judgment that the hospice notion is not one that can be easily contained once a commitment is made to it. Those hospitals planning hospices without inpatient facilities (and these currently make up nine out of ten hospitals involved in hospice planning) are likely to find themselves with a continuing issue that must sooner or later be resolved at the highest policy levels.

Finally, we ask our clients if all the nuances of reimbursement are understood—Medicare, Medicaid, Title 20, and Older Americans Act. These programs are potential financial sources for hospice services, but a number of potential hospice patients are not eligible for any of the four. There are also limits to what can be done for those who are eligible. Emotional support services, most homemaker services, and even bereavement followup do not appear to be reimbursable.

If a new reimbursement source were developed and Congress approved hospice as a separate service, the dollar situation would change. However, so would many other elements in the equation, such as strict directions and regulations affecting services and organizations and limits on hospital sponsorship.

We tell our clients that the hope for a useful and successful program may be justified only if the hospital has considered all these questions and only if they appreciate how truly new and untested all hospice approaches are—particularly those in an acute care hospital setting.

25

A Physical Alternative to the Hospice

Lo-Yi Chan

The answer to what a physical alternative to a hospice might look like can be found in a newspaper's classified ads: "Paneled living room, paneled dining room, wood-burning fireplace, river view." Here too, continuing care might be given.

Is this absurd? If someone has uremia, how can such luxury help? In talking about a continuum of care, perhaps we should also be talking about a continuum of environment. It is absurd to say that I can translate an apartment overlooking the Hudson River in New York City to the 19th floor of a large medical center. Yet some things might be possible.

The proposition is very simple. The most effective use of our potential space is found only in an environment that enables both patient and family to live effectively in the face of impending death.

A large acute-care hospital has many goals—care, cure, economy, efficiency, safety, research, and education. These goals may often be mutually exclusive, but they are generally accepted and shared by most people involved with any one of them and even by the patients who lose a lot to stay alive. The patients suffer a loss of privacy and in many cases loss of self-determination. Under a hospital-based continuing care service, all goals should be subservient to the environment that enables patients and family to live effectively in the face of impending death. How can a medical center, teaching hospital do this?

First, look at the patient. We found in thinking about the hospice in Connecticut that patients near death need support to maintain a stable concept of self. They face many unknowns. They are losing control of their degenerating bodies. Some of this focuses on their environment, for perhaps, they cannot move around very much. They lose perception. Therefore, the environment has two opposing goals: to develop a sense of privacy so that the patient can maintain that sense of self and to create a sense of community so that the patient can have support from around him. We are talking about living rooms and dining rooms and continuing the business of everyday living for the patient and family.

Space needs are the needs for space in everyday activities: living, shopping, going out of doors. These can be "destination" spaces, and it could be possible for a large hospital to make room for them. Patients could go down to a gift shop. A coffee shop should not be a little hole in the wall. It should have a large flashing neon sign that says, "coffee," and the patient might have that as a goal.

I remember seeing a totally paralyzed patient in a Massachusetts hospital. Every day she would put on all her clothes, including her shoes, and just lie in bed. That was her outing for the day. How much better to take a patient, fully clothed, in bed, right down to the coffee shop. A service needs a variety of spaces that come closer to the patient's life style, not just spaces for sleeping and medication.

In order for this space to enable patients to live effectively, we must get closer to working with families. In many ways the families are more important to the environment than the patients are because the family is so much more aware of the environment. They see more cues than the patient because some patients are comatose and some are letting go. Often the first thing they let go of is the environment. Families are full of anxiety—there are all kinds of unknowns for them. The facility can help them best by easing anxiety.

In the Connecticut Hospice we have created anterooms—spaces that lead to other spaces so that one does not confront anything directly. It sounds rather difficult, but it is fairly easy because a typical hospital has all kinds of space requirements. We use some of these spaces to lead to other spaces.

In an apartment you do not open the door, walk in, and see the bedroom. You go through the foyer, the living room, and maybe a hall. Isn't that logical for a family who visits the patient in a hospital? If a visitor is not a close family member, it is even more important to have this sequence of spaces to reach the patient.

Another group of people is the staff, professional staff, as well as volunteer. They have very different conflicting requirements: a need to take action and a need to retreat. Fortunately, staff are more mobile than families and the patients, and those environments can be made easily available in a hospital. The point is that one has to want to do it. Most hospitals have space for action; they don't have space for retreat, and so the staff find these on their own. They use the nurses' station and hide behind all the papers and files for retreat. Perhaps the design should be that a retreat is really a retreat, and when a nurse or other staff members are there, they are permitted to retreat. In turn, it may mean that when they are in a place where they can act (that is, the bedside), they will more likely act.

What does all this mean to the hospital in general? We are really dealing with people. Despite all of the technology, the egos, and symptoms and diseases, in the end we are still talking about physical environments that give comfort.

26

A Psychiatric Setting and Total Care

Samuel C. Klagsbrun

Professors of the old school of psychology believed that if a small area in a frame of reference is changed, the relationship of the entirety will be changed. Unlike scientific speculation about specific variables, this disregards any concept of specific variables in terms of relationship to the whole. In changing a setting such as that of geriatric centers or a unit in a general hospital to a free-standing hospice, good care can be delivered to dying patients and their families with resources not previously thought of.

At Four Winds Hospital in Katonah, New York, much has occurred in innovative, nonplanned ways that supports this change. It was decided that the Four Winds be called a psychiatric hospital and that the entire staff and facility be geared toward the psychiatric setting—to talking, sharing, expressing, and to long-term care and commitment. Although I believe in a community of people as a basis for hospice care, I am a psychiatrist who is also interested in the physical science of medical care.

The first patient eligible for hospice care at Four Winds was a young woman with a psychiatric history that, perhaps, made her unplaceable in another kind of facility. She was a bright, 24-year-old individual who had entered Four Winds with cancer. When Betsy came to us, I had had the idea of opening Four Winds to hospice care. Betsy was referred because she was a psychiatric patient who happened to be dying and because I was a psychiatrist in a hospital that was looking into hospice care.

Betsy was ambulatory at admission. We did worry about the impact she would have on the psychiatric patients. What would a schizophrenic patient feel in group therapy with a dying patient? What about a middle-aged depressive, who had entered the hospital to deal with losses, sitting in a group with a person who was experiencing the loss of her life? What effect would it have on the hospital atmosphere and on the staff? Yet what better time could there be to seize opportunities that dying patients give us when they are ready to talk or share or need support?

We have all kinds of professional people who respond quickly, effectively, and immediately to any communication from a patient facing death, and we were able to offer pain control and management on a medical level for this patient. We watched interaction and were absolutely amazed at what we learned. We let experience teach us rather than conceptualize ahead of time. The schizophrenic patients as a group suddenly seemed to gain philosophical perspectives on their difficulties. It was fascinating to watch Jack, the young man who had been deeply psychotic for a long, long time, try to offer Betsy something. Betsy, totally lost in her own sense of loss, gave Jack a hard time. It was not so easy to reach her. Somehow, the entire place started to see Betsy as a bit of a challenge. They did not see her as a dying patient for whom psychosocial death takes place before death. They saw her as someone to whom they could offer a part of themselves because she was dying. That kind of impact on our psychiatric population could never have been predicted.

Betsy lived for three months in a rather remarkable way and participated in activities to the extent that she was able. From St. Christopher's Hospice (London) I learned that no patient wants to be a prisoner in his own bed simply because the bed is not on wheels and the door is too narrow. So we prepared a bed on wheels that could navigate through every doorway. It was not unusual to have Betsy, even toward the end of her time, participate in a group activity with others. Everyone else would be sitting, and Betsy would lie on her stomach on the rolling bed.

Because she was in a psychiatric setting, Betsy would talk in a psychiatric fashion. She expressed her feelings of loss and her bitterness. In this kind of atmosphere (perhaps contrary to that in an acute medical ward that is being changed into a hospice), rage, outrageous behavior, terrible language, and awkward vocabulary are taken for granted. The staff encourages expressions of emotions.

Betsy taught us about the real needs of patients. She reminded me that in medical centers providing hospice care, our colleagues are often not trained in psychiatry. They may often question the patient in a language or tone that does not necessarily invite communication. The wave of a hand and a "how are you" are not really invitations to talk or to share. But if one sits on the edge of the bed and holds a patient's hand, one indicates that one is not going to move unless the patient says something that is real. A psychiatric setting lends itself to more communication possibilities than a busy, otherwise occupied center does.

Betsy taught us that there is a moment when it is time to die. After her experiences of intense and lively moments with the group, she announced to the staff and the group in many different ways that it was time to say goodbye. On one occasion she did say that she would no longer participate in any activities in the hospital and retreated to her room. Although we tried to change her mind, she never emerged from that room.

In the room was another bed we had deliberately provided for family or for anyone else who wanted to stay. Unfortunately, for Betsy, existing family relationships and involvement were not available. This could have been detrimental. However, the extra bed in Betsy's room was often shared by one who was there on her invitation—her beautiful Irish setter. Upon admission to the hospital, Betsy had given one condition: that her dog be allowed anywhere in the hospital along with her and have access to any place, including sleeping under her bed (much to the concern of the housekeeping department). This wonderful, beautiful dog was permitted to sleep with Betsy even at the time she was saying goodbye to us.

At the end of her time, Betsy controlled the circle of people permitted into her room. As her horizon diminished, the number of people whom she allowed to be with her also shrank. We all understood that. In group discussion, she was endlessly the topic of discussion. People in the hospital to take care of their depressions understood Betsy and respected what she was doing. When one is very depressed, one does not want to be bothered with too many stimuli. On some level, one does want to be left alone. Sometimes it is important to allow that, sometimes it is important to challenge it.

Betsy died at Four Winds. Our biggest problem then was what to do with the dog. We all wanted a piece of Betsy to remain with us; we wanted that dog. For many reasons, we felt that the family did not deserve to have Betsy's dog, and we actually got into a battle over this legacy. At the same moment in my role as medical director, I decided we would have to mourn our loss and allow the dog to return to the family. A "Lassie-come-home" story ensued; the dog came back to us. I regret to say we returned it to the family.

What we had learned from this one experience opened the entire hospital, including patients, friends, and relatives of patients, to the possibility of allowing Four Winds to move into hospice care. We have continued this on a very modest level with one or two patients who have come to Four Winds to live until they die.

From experience, we have learned that many physical details can be worried about after the fact instead of ahead of time. If one opens areas that one never thought about before in terms of hospice care, one may find there are people who can handle these situations. They succeed better when acting spontaneously than if preplanning systems or approaches had been established, although some system and preparation are necessary to embark on this adventure.

Ultimately, hospice care ends up being people care. A small group of people make the commitment to giving *total care* to the patient and the family. They can be constantly available without any bureaucratic barriers.

If one has enough people who know the personal demands made upon staff, and enough who have the correct kind of energy, one is prepared. Other systems might lend themselves to experimenting in hospice—communal towns, communes located in rural areas where the community is much more integrated than in a large city. There are certainly opportunities in nursing homes, old age homes, and senior citizen programs that lend themselves to hospice care. And there are other directions that are potentially exciting to think about. We should experiment with changing some of the parts around to see how they fit into a whole that will help us achieve our goals.

27

Caring for the Terminally Ill: The Story of an American Hospital

James E. Cimino

Calvary Hospital has been involved in the care of terminally ill patients since 1899, when a group of Catholic laywomen in lower New York City dedicated their lives to caring for patients who were indigent and near death. Over the years Calvary, which originally treated any seriously ill or dying patient, has evolved into an advanced-cancer hospital. It has always maintained the tradition of treating those who could not pay. In 1915, the people who began this program moved it into a private home in the Bronx. It is now located directly across from the Albert Einstein College of Medicine.

In the past, it was never clear as to whether Calvary was a nursing home, an acute-care facility, or a chronic-care hospital. Its nursing staff was a group of highly motivated, dedicated Catholic sisters. The attendance of the medical staff was rather erratic; sometimes there was difficulty finding a physician to pronounce a patient dead. The indications for admission to the hospital were not clearly defined. The waiting list was so large that it was exasperating for social workers who wanted to refer patients.

In recent years, the waiting lists have become shorter. On some days they are nonexistent. This is a credit to the hospice movement's impact. If Calvary did not exist we would not be missed in the same way we would have been before 1975, because it is now difficult to find an institution of any credibility that does not have some people intensely interested in caring for rather than abandoning the terminally ill patient.

In 1965, Calvary applied for and obtained official recognition from the Joint Commission on Accreditation of Hospitals. This has attracted greater public funding and has enabled its large deficit to be reduced. Formerly, only indigent people were admitted. These people now receive benefits under the Medicare/Medicaid laws, and for the most part proper reimbursement is made to the hospital.

At the present time, Calvary is at a turning point. The nursing order of Catholic sisters who had been so intimately involved in the program until 1973 began to do things other than dedicate their entire lives to Calvary Hospital. The sisters worked seven days a week and 16 to 17 hours a day. They lived on the premises and were able to inspire everyone around them, including physicians. Before and during my 1961 affiliation at Calvary, I was involved in many activities. By 1970, I abandoned my other interests for the work there. Other physicians also left their practices and came to Calvary full time.

Until the mid-1970s, Calvary Hospital had virtually no employee turnover. People would inquire about our staff support program. We had no formal program. We did not even have a sense of formal team management, although the management was there because everyone involved was consulted. Most people working at the hospital were happy, although Calvary is not the kind of place one would expect to provide a positive environment. Many years ago it had the reputation of being a death house; children and others would avoid walking past it. But it certainly is not like that.

Calvary is sponsored by the New York Catholic Archdiocese, but we have people of many denominations on our staff, and we consider them all important members of our program. Since a move into new facilities, which has increased its capacity from 111 beds to a potential for 200 beds, Calvary has had to add a tremendous number of staff. It has had problems with new people, partly because they were not certain what Calvary was. Unfortunately, some of the people interested in the hospice movement who have come to work at Calvary are very intense and uncompromising when they believe that our program falters. Some have not worked out their own difficulties with physicians and with the whole social order of medicine.

In order to enter Calvary, a patient should have a physician's honest appraisal of a short life expectancy. That is not easy to predict. We ask that a guess of prognosis for two to six weeks of life be made, although that figure is becoming artificial. The original reason for this requirement was that the sisters wanted to care for as many of the dying as possible.

We do have empty beds, and we are looking for slightly longer term patients. However, our designation as an acute-care hospital and our struggle with utilization and peer review create many difficulties. We want people who are very sick. The paradox is that we provide what we consider high-quality medical, nursing, social work, pastoral care, and recreation therapy. But very often the best of all of this appears to our reviewers as though it is unnecessary.

Those involved in this field know otherwise. Visiting a patient three or four times a day is very therapeutic, in spite of the fact that anticancer medications may be withdrawn. We have no standard policies on the management of the patient other than our philosophy of compassionate care, symptom relief, and "non-abandonment." Calvary patients can be given IVs, chemotherapy, radiation and very occasional surgical procedures. We attempt to offer the patient and family not only what we think is the best care but also what they would like to have. We are not dictatorial in presenting the kind of care that we give. Of the patients admitted, 50 percent die within 30 days and 75 percent within 60 days. Our physicians do not always correctly guess the life expectancy of a patient.

We have no policy about informing patients that they have cancer nor of informing them of their prognoses. We do not confront the patient with this information. However, if the patient and the family appear to be having difficulties or if decisions have to be made in management (including withdrawal of therapy) that they are resisting, we will discuss these issues honestly with both the patient and the family.

As a rule, I question patients on admission and encourage them into saying why they think they are at the hospital. Very often they say it is because they are sick. I ask them what they are sick from, and they will say that they really do not know. I ask further and say, "Well, you have a scar on your abdomen. What happened? Did you have an operation? What did they find?" I want to know what the doctor told them. Depending on how the patient takes the lead, I either pursue further or let the matter drop. Some patients have come to us with the truth and all the facts known.

Patients or families with preconceived notions about progressive stages of death and dying are often the very people who require the most attention and patience. They often are the most difficult to manage. We once received a patient from another hospital with the resident's diagnosis of "malignancy, end stage, Kübler-Ross' stage three." Although we give credit to Kübler-Ross' work, we ourselves are not very accepting of staging. Even she would agree that stages are not clearcut, are transient, and that there are many substages.

Over the years we have tried not to deny the patients access to any kind of of care they think appropriate. We do not treat under protocol studies unless they are nontoxic and then only in cooperation with one of the larger medical centers. Of our nine attending physicians (every patient is assigned an internist), only one can be considered an oncologist, and he does not do much oncology per se. We have had many oncologists come through our medical staff. Some have provided coverage for various periods of time, but none have remained with us. That has always told us something: medical oncologists must find this kind of work extremely frustrating.

Why do this work? I am almost embarrassed to answer. It makes me feel good to know that I am helping someone at the most difficult time of his life. What is the other alternative? Why have we not written more about ourselves? How do we talk about being a Good Samaritan? It's all been said. We have no magic.

I believe that if dying is acknowledged by an individual, whether it is acceptance or resignation, it is usually because he expects something better. I wonder how someone can go out of this life peacefully believing that there is nothing to follow. Those who have real conviction about what is waiting for them and feel that there is a future life will also be in a quandary about where they are going. If they believe they are going "up," they will go out happily. If they believe that they are not, they will depart with a struggle. We have not made any keen observations about the death of religious people, and we have not noticed that people who are trained in religion and philosophy seem to die happier than others. Patients who know the most about their illness very often appear to have a more difficult time. Dr. Raimbault, a French psychiatrist, categorized patients on a medical oncology service as having good or bad deaths. Raimbault reported that patients who had difficult deaths were often those whose chemotherapy had been discontinued a long time before death; who knew the most about their illnesses; and who were exposed to conflicts among staff members or frequent staff changes.

In my experience, "teaching hospitals" rarely give patients with poor prognoses excellent care. On a teaching service with young people interested in gaining knowledge, it is more difficult to give these patients the appropriate attention.

We do not have a home care service, although we hope to. Over the years, we have not had to address the home situation because most of our patients did not have a suitable home environment and many did not even have families.

In conclusion, the services that a hospice wishes to provide require competent, emotionally mature, compassionate people who can be available to the patient or family at any time. These caregivers must not be individuals who are attempting to work out their own problems with facing death or grief. Their attendance must be strong, objective, and sensitive, and it must focus on the needs of the patient. Those already involved in this work know the satisfactions and the burdens of their efforts. Success in this field has always been due to the ability to attract inspired, hardworking people with, more often than not, religious zeal and conviction. The cold reality is that these people are in very short supply. How hospices or any health service can continue to attract such people should be a major concern now and for the future.

28

Integrating Care for the Terminally Ill Within a Comprehensive Geriatric Center

William Liss-Levinson

When examining the history of the hospice movement in America, one is struck by the rapid development of this new member of the health care delivery system. The Connecticut Hospice, the first in the United States, began providing services in 1971. Currently, estimates on the number of hospices being planned range from 200 to 400 and about 100 are operational. The recognition of problems inherent both in health care institutions and in the nature of the delivery system itself has sparked this almost charismatic drive to improve the quality of caring for terminally ill persons and their family members.

The Development of Hospice in New York State

New York State recognized the need to establish legislation to certify this new type of health care as a legitimate member of the health care system. On August 7, 1978, Governor Hugh Carey signed into law a bill that established hospice demonstration projects. The focus of this demonstration program was twofold: to determine if hospice care is a high-quality alternative to traditional health care services offered to the terminally ill and to assess the relative cost-effectiveness of hospice care. These programs, implemented in January 1980 for a three-year period, are to be the basis for (intended) eventual licensure of hospices throughout the state. The law also emphasized the importance of home care, with three models of backup inpatient beds:

a) in an autonomous unit of a hospital or nursing care facility
b) in a free-standing hospice unit
c) in whatever unit of a hospital the patient is admitted to (sometimes referred to as a "scattered-bed" hospice).

The Public Health Council, charged with responsibility for establishing the demonstration programs, selected 15 programs throughout the state. The actual management of the program became the responsibility of the Office of Health Systems Management's Bureau of Health Maintenance Organizations (HMO) and Home Health Care. One such designated program is The Brooklyn Hospice at Metropolitan Jewish Geriatric Center.

Hospice as Part of a Geriatric Center: A Rationale

It is understandable why a hospital, which daily deals with terminal illness, issues of palliation, and symptom control would be an ideal institution in which to develop a hospice program. Equally, a certified home health agency, which is already skilled in the maintenance of patients at home, is a logical choice for a hospice program. A geriatric nursing care facility may, however, seem a somewhat puzzling setting for hospice care. On the one hand, given the average age of residents, a geriatric center is already working with a population who (from an actuarial standpoint) are close to death. However, most could not be considered terminal, as defined by the state hospital code, subchapter C of chapter V of title 10, section 790.1 (b) "A person in the terminal stage of illness, with a life expectancy of approximately six months or less." Furthermore, the average geriatric facility generally does not have staff with expertise in symptom control, palliation, and psychosocial support for the terminally ill and bereaved, which is essential to the functioning of a hospice program.

To address these issues and thus understand the promise of Metropolitan Jewish Geriatric Center's (MJGC) Brooklyn Hospice, we must first examine MJGC as a comprehensive geriatric center.

Metropolitan Jewish Geriatric Center

History

Established in 1907 as the Brooklyn Hebrew Home and Hospital for the Aged, this voluntary nonprofit, nonsectarian institution has become one of the nation's leading health care institutions serving chronically ill and disabled adults. Its inpatient facilities consist of a 529-bed skilled nursing facility (SNF) and a 386-bed health-related facility (HRF). At both these facilities (approved by the Joint Commission on American Hospitals) a total of 915 persons can receive the most up-to-date care services, which include the following:

- round-the-clock physician services
- 24-hour nursing care
- access to a 19-bed maximum care unit
- direct access to a major medical center
- psychiatric treatment
- social services
- nutritional consultation and services
- physical therapy
- occupational therapy
- recreational therapy
- speech therapy
- pastoral support and services
- a variety of specialty medical care services.

Service to the Community

MJGC's firm commitment to discovering improved ways for maintaining the independence and life satisfaction of older adults has resulted
in the development of a number of innovative programs designed to
keep people out of institutions. The Center's day hospital program
provides a variety of health care services (medical, rehabilitative, psychosocial, and recreational) to elderly persons and thus enables them to
remain at home in the community. The long-term home health care
program offers a coordinated plan of care for people who are homebound and who would otherwise require institutionalization. An emergency alarm response system has been implemented that enables the
elderly to receive emergency help in times of crises. Future plans call
for a rehabilitation unit, mobile geriatric screening team, self-care
health education project, and other programs that emphasize prevention,
diagnosis, restoration, and maintenance. This emphasis on community
service, and particularly on programs that help keep elderly people with
health problems out of institutions by creating alternatives, is one of the
sources of MJGC's interest in hospice.

Additionally, an analysis of mortality rates, patient care, and institutional utilization trends in the borough of Brooklyn disclosed one of
the highest cancer death rates in the state. Moreover, the investigation
pointed to glaring gaps in the health care delivery system for terminally
ill patients and their families. A review of the patient population in
hospices in the United States, Canada, and Great Britain indicated that
the vast majority of hospice patients could be expected to be 60 years of
age and over. Thus, the potential patient population would generally not
be foreign to the institution.

Jewish Tradition and the Hospice Concept

Communal involvement in the care of the sick, especially the incurably
ill, has a long history in Jewish cultural life. Moreover, care from the
Jewish perspective has always been designed to provide spiritual, social,
and emotional support, as well as needed medical attention. Hospice as

a philosophy and modality of care is, thus, compatible both with Jewish religious and cultural tradition and with MJGC's long-standing mission of service to the community.

While admission to the center and its programs is not restricted for reasons of race, religious orientation, national origin, sponsor, or handicap, the facility does observe Orthodox Jewish dietary and religious laws (monitored by a resident rabbi), and Jewish tradition and practices play a major role in shaping the program's compassionate approach to death and bereavement. This makes the center's program one of the first to be operated under Jewish auspices.

Concern with the emotional welfare of the terminally ill, as expressed by Kübler-Ross and other thanatologists, is not new to Judaism. Jewish tradition has long considered the needs of the dying person and his family, as well as the therapeutic value of grieving. It is a tradition that enables people to reaffirm life's meaning and strengthen family and community ties. The Brooklyn Hospice can draw on the humane lessons detailed in Jewish law to maintain the emotional equilibrium of the terminal patient and his family. Jewish tradition in conjunction with modern psychological insights can provide a framework for dealing with the mourning, grief, and despair of surviving loved ones and with the challenge of reintegrating them into the community of living.

Metropolitan's unique history and philosophy of caring, coupled with its diverse institutional and community-based programs, make it an excellent setting for a hospice program that incorporates the various programs together with services of a specially trained team of health care professionals.

Staffing

In order to offer the range of care services necessary to a hospice program, the hospice staff is composed of a team of various health care professionals. Underlying these individuals' personal and professional qualifications is a deep commitment to the hospice philosophy of caring. Coupled with this is also a realistic and emotionally healthy awareness of personal strengths and limitations—a vital quality for health care professionals working in a highly stressful environment.

In addition to the hospice director (a psychologist with experience in counseling the terminally ill and bereaved and in training and supervision), the following professionals constitute the hospice team:

> physician-in-chief
> physician's assistant
> patient care coordinator (Master's level nurse)
> chief social worker
> coordinator of volunteer services
> pastoral care coordinator
> education and consultation coordinator
> recreation therapists
> nursing personnel

This interdisciplinary approach to patient care, combined with the knowledge and expertise of consultants in the areas of oncology, psychiatry, radiology, pharmacology, dentistry, physical therapy, and dietetics, enables the hospice to reach out to the diverse needs of patients and their families. Also, these professionals bring to the team a variety of personal and professional orientations and styles that help facilitate learning, growth, and mutual support.

Program Aims and Methods of Implementation

Dedicated to safeguarding the quality of life for those suffering from irreversible illnesses, the Brooklyn Hospice is a coordinated program of in-home, outpatient, and institutional care. It offers a diversity of supportive services by an interdisciplinary team of sensitive and highly skilled professionals, paraprofessionals, and trained volunteers. All persons in need of care will be served without regard to race, religious orientation, national origin, age, sex, or sponsor.

The majority of patients—forty at any given time—are cared for at home. Nursing care, physician visits, and psychosocial and spiritual support are all provided to enable the individual to remain at home until death or as long as possible (and desired). Volunteers play a vital role in the home care program, both providing direct patient support (emotional and/or recreational) and enabling family members to have a respite from their caring responsibilities.

It is anticipated that approximately 60 percent of the patients (25) on the home care program would be able to come one or two times a week to the center's day hospital. This provides them with an opportunity to have a change of environment, socialize and interact with other people, receive various institutionally based services; and become familiar with staff and layout of the inpatient unit.

Those patients requiring more intensive medical attention are cared for in a home-like continuing care unit. This 10-bed unit attempts to create an atmosphere maximizing the positive aspects of dying at home while providing for the more intensive medical and nursing needs of the patient. Liberal visitation policies enable both patient and family to interact and share in the dying process as they would at home. Special attention to dietary needs and the full range of services provided at home are also available here. Volunteers are also used in a variety of ways to maximize support to the patient and his family.

Also concerned with the higher rate of illness, hospitalization, and premature death among recently bereaved individuals, as well as with obstacles to social reintegration confronted by widowed persons, the Brooklyn Hospice is committed to a program of followup care for families during the bereavement period. Individual and group counseling and therapy, visitation and telephone reassurance, annual death remembrances, social services, and legal assistance are provided for up to one year following the death of the patient.

Education and Consultation Services

In addition to direct patient and family services, the Brooklyn Hospice recognizes that many professionals and laypersons lack basic information regarding the needs of terminally ill persons. The hospice has a commitment to serve as a community resource for the dissemination of information about terminal illnesses, death, dying, loss, and bereavement. The education and consultation coordinator develops workshops and seminars geared to the specific needs of such groups as physicians, nurses, social workers, clergypersons, and the lay community.

Other plans call for a newsletter to relate the latest research findings and advancements in the care of the terminally ill to the professional community, a toll-free number for information and referral, a consultation service to instruct health care personnel in the latest pharmacological and nonpharmacological techniques in pain management and symptom control, a central depository containing relevant literature and audiovisual materials, and the development of brochures, pamphlets, and guidebooks for professional and lay use.

Reimbursement and Financing of the Hospice Program

The problems confronting the issue of reimbursement for hospice care services in the United States are too complex for inclusion in this article. The geriatric center does maintain a strong commitment to using its own funds, in combination with philanthropic and grant monies, and various third-party reimbursement mechanisms.

Summary

The future of hospice care in America depends on the ability of health care institutions and professionals to see beyond their four walls, beyond the scope of the traditional health care delivery system. Bold, brave steps must be taken to realize the goal of helping people to truly live until they die. Metropolitan Jewish Geriatric Center is one pioneer in this area.

Postscript

There is an old Yiddish saying, *A mensch tracht, un gut lacht*—"a person thinks and plans, and G-d laughs." When this article was written, it was the author's expectation that the Hospice program it describes would be fully implemented. However, reimbursement for Hospice services has not been established, and the Metropolitan Jewish Geriatric Center has had to alter the scope of The Brooklyn Hospice and its services.

In the area of staffing, in addition to the Director, the Hospice employs the following: a Medical Director, Chief Social Worker, Education and Consultation Coordinator, a Nurse Coordinator, and a Social Work Coordinator (with responsibility for screening and intake and the Volunteer component). The plan for a discrete ten-bed, inpatient unit has never been realized. Existing reimbursement available at the Skilled Nursing Facility inpatient rate would not cover even half the cost of operating an inpatient unit, as was envisioned. Patients cared for at home by the Hospice program, for whom home care is no longer feasible, have been admitted on a selected basis to the Skilled Nursing Facility. While the Hospice team continues their intensive and extensive intervention with said patient and family, the level of nursing care is no different from that provided for any other resident in the facility.

The average monthly caseload is between 20 to 25 patient/families, generally consisting of ten to twelve home care cases; three to five counseling cases (in situations where the patient has not been on the Hospice program); and seven bereavement follow-up cases (since only about one-half of families serviced desire and/or require ongoing formal bereavement counseling from the Hospice in the year follow-up period).

The type of patient referred to the program has also generally not been ambulatory or transportable for involvement in the Center's Day Hospital program as we initially envisioned. Finally, while the Education and Consultation Services have been extensive and a clear means of reaching out (ultimately) to a far larger population than we could serve directly, certain of the proposed components have never been developed. Specifically, the newsletter and the toll-free information number have never been implemented. It should be noted, however, that the Hospice staff nonetheless provides information and referrals to approximately 20 to 25 callers per month who are not appropriate for admission to the Hospice program.

Surviving through grants, philanthropic funds, and family donations, The Brooklyn Hospice has managed to evolve into a viable (albeit limited) service program for the terminally ill. Hospice as a health care phenomenon has grown rapidly. There are at this time over 450 operational programs in the United States, and recent estimates by the Joint

Commission on the Accreditation of Hospitals (JCAH) are that an additional 360 programs are in the planning stage. Legislation to amend existing Medicare regulations to include Hospice care services was passed by the Congress and signed by President Reagan in September 1982. When implemented, in mid-1983, it will represent a boon not only to The Brooklyn Hospice and other operational hospices, but also will allow for the continued growth and development of Hospice programs to truly meet the needs of the terminally ill of this country. Thus, while tempered by the realities of our past experiences, we look to the future with optimism and a renewed spirit of commitment to help ease the pain of death.

29

Dying and Death of a Hospice in a Tertiary Hospital: Case History

Peter G. Wilson

New York Hospital has always been known as a tertiary hospital and acute treatment center. With increasing financial difficulties and a review board, patients who are dying could not well stay within our system, nor did we want them, unless extreme diversionary tactics could be used, such as putting the patients on a waiting list for placement in a "home"—which we know would take a long time. These patients would have to be moved out. A number of concerned internists and surgeons who had worked with their patients over a long stretch of time found this increasingly onerous and began meeting informally trying to find out what they could do about keeping their dying patients in this hospital. In addition, the patients' families—very distressed by this kind of procedure—were beginning to write nasty letters to the administration, causing considerable noxious stimulation. Two further fortuitous circumstances occurred. A wealthy patient died rather miserably over a longish period of time, and he and his family decided to set up a foundation that could look at this problem within the hospital. With this money two "prophets" were imported, one from London and one from Montreal, in order to raise the consciousness of the medical center. To these meetings came primarily medical students and junior staff members, plus a number of the highest echelon staff members. The middle-echelon people in most departments seemed to stay away. Also, a grant possibility emerged and gave the strongest push to get the process going.

The administrative posture was that this sounded like a marvelous idea, that certainly the grant proposal should go in. With the willingness of one of the large departments to supply some space (which is at a premium), the honeymoon period was in full swing.

Opening Phase

A committee was formed made up of two groups of people. One group was composed of doctors who had originally felt that they needed space for their patients to die appropriately and a social worker and nurse who were willing to do the leg work in terms of getting the grant in. A second group of people on the committee had an interest in the hospice—a chaplain, an oncologist, and a psychiatrist—and were brought in for their particular expertise. Since action had to be started on two fronts—get the grant in and start working through community boards to have beds allocated for a hospice—the administration sent people around who would be willing to look at how expensive it would be to the hospital and to the community in terms of beds.

Some hard issues had to be faced, and quickly the honeymoon period between the committee and the administration began taking on some darker hues. As examples: it became obvious that there would be some loss of individual bed money to the hospital; that even with the money from the demonstration project, most of the physicians—both voluntary and full time—would have to work "free"; and that some basic changes in architecture of a unit would have to be made within the hospital setting.

Middle Phase: Dying

At this time the grant proposal had been submitted, and time had to be spent with the community boards on a city level. Two of the most active part-time, voluntary people were carrying most of the fight at tremendous cost to them, but there was obvious progress as one approval after the other came through. The first grant indications were supposed to come through, and weekly telephone calls to Washington were instituted to find out what was happening.

The committee continued to meet, one of the major problems being committee morale. The meetings dealt with possible grant money, and there was a distinct split of the committee into two groups—one saying that we absolutely needed this money to set up an appropriate unit that could be properly staffed up to proper scientific standards and proper patient care, and a second group that began saying that it would be just as well if we did not get the grant because this demonstration grant would demand that we show results within 2½ years, and we were not sure we could do it. The committee was split about 50/50 on this.

The committee kept the administration apprised of what was happening and indeed needed many letters for city and state agencies and for the federal grant, which the administration seemed happy to supply. All in all it was a very quiet time and the administration in essence said nothing.

Late Middle Phase: Dying

At this time the city and state battles had been won. The approval for the conversion of the beds was in, and news of final grant support was about four months late. As far as the committee was concerned, it was felt that whether we got the money or not we would need some "standards" of admission and an administrative structure. The committee was still split among the same two groups. The group that had hopes for getting the money became representative of a "large" number of beds (12), and the group that would have been just as happy not to get the grant wanted very few beds (3-4) so that we could feel our way along. The group who wanted a small number of beds naturally began thinking of rules of admission that would keep people out, while the ones who wanted more beds tended to be overinclusive and dealt mainly with how to keep people within the system.

The administration, now that they were faced with approval from the city and state agencies, began having serious second thoughts about allocating the beds and went on record with their serious reservations. Although money was said to be the root of the reservations, the whole idea of having a hospice within the hospital seemed to be a hard reality to deal with.

Death and Resurrection?

The news came through that we had not been awarded a grant. The committee was devastated, the larger group feeling that without this money it was impossible to go on. The smaller group felt that it was just as well and that we should go on anyway. The administration now felt that there was good reason to table the project and, in an ironic twist, the medical board appointed an official hospice committee while the project had been quietly buried by the administration.

Out of this wreckage the committee decided to form a roving band that like other roving bands—oncology, kidney, hypertension—would make itself available on a consultative basis and, more than that, would search out situations where we might be of help. This is where we are at the present time.

These facts can be looked at in a slightly different way by using the concepts of denial, anger, bargaining, depression, and acceptance.

First, looking at it from the position of the administration, death and dying were topics that had not been dealt with, and it was strongly felt that they should not be dealt with. Denial was strong, and the willingness to touch this material minimal. At the beginning, when money became "available," the administration was really forced into the position of looking at this unsavory topic. From the beginning, the administration was angry at the committee for even bringing these concepts up, but the anger was never dealt with by the committee in the fear that dealing with it would show us the true torrential, angry nature and the administration would then refuse to go any further. The administration did provide two people to look at the financial status and to help with seeing how much money it would cost, and this was interpreted by the committee as an attempt to work with them and cooperate in a difficult situation. An alternative hypothesis is that this was part of the denial of the problem, dealing with the mechanical money problems as a way of not dealing with death, that is, like the patient who, when informed that he is dying, goes into a flurry of activity in setting up a will, making sure that there is adequate money for his family, telling his family where the money is, but not dealing with the fact in regard to himself or the family that there is a terminal point. It could also be seen in the sense of bargaining in that if they gave the committee some help, we would then stop bugging them about the whole concept—death, dying, and hospices.

As a counterpoint to this, it would be profitable to look at the two groups within the committee: group 1, who had been the original movers who needed space for their patients plus a social worker and a nurse; and group 2, the people who had an intellectual or an emotional stake but came primarily as representatives of their departments. Group 1 had worked through many of their defenses in standing at the abyss with their patients, had worked through some of their depression, and were obviously accepting the difficulties of what was to come—death. Group 2, on the other hand, coming from a more theoretical base and not intimately involved, were set up for the denial, anger, and bargaining that had not been worked through. In some ways it seems obvious that this group, in unconscious collusion with the administration, accentuated many of the difficulties that came later.

By the middle phase, while the administration was being quiet, the assumption was made by the committee that the interest had continued and that if they fought the good fight, the administration would indeed back them. There were small glints of hope in that when the committee asked for some letters of support, they were forthcoming. But it could be argued that since no pressure was being exerted for something more, the denial could remain as strong as ever. As far as the committee was concerned, the smaller group, saying that we could do with less and probably should, seemed to have picked up fairly early that their position was an unpopular one and unlikely to attract the powers of the hospital, medical school, and government. Therefore, the issues that should be dealt with were the nuts and bolts of how to set up even a small seed that could sprout slowly. The larger group, on the other hand, were not aware of how hot and unpopular an issue they were dealing with. Their own denial was probably equally strong, and their anger in bargaining with both the government and the hospital administration was an attempt not to deal with their own feelings of helplessness and omnipotence vis-à-vis death.

In the late middle stage, in the time when the governmental agencies had given their approval for the setting up of a hospice and we had not yet been turned down in regard to the grant, the administration suddenly woke up to the fact that they would have to deal with the real situation. God forbid that the money would come through—this might have caused all kinds of problems. At this point they made it very clear that they had severe reservations, and it was equally clear that they wished the committee would just go away. The anger at having to be faced with this kind of a decision was very obvious, and the hospital's not getting the grant effectively closed the door to the problem. Once again they did not have to face the question of a hospice.

As far as the committee was concerned, the smaller group was able to take this pretty much in stride, in some ways saying "I told you so" and could begin thinking of alternative plans while keeping the issue alive. The larger group, not having faced the difficulty of the situation, now could become extremely depressed—as they did—and it is now a question of whether they will be able to work this through toward some kind of acceptance of the difficulty and unpopularity of the cause they espoused or go back to isolation and denial.

The bottom line is that this is a difficult topic that, when brought to the attention of hospital administration, is fought in similar a way to that of the patient who finds out he is dying. This may be worked through toward some kind of a status where one accepts the limitations and difficulties, or one can continue to deny them. In our experience, the administration continued to deny as, unfortunately, did the members of the larger group, whose insistence on the power of upwardly mobile, "living" issues may have helped in buttressing the administration's position.

30

Hospice Home Care

Robert W. Buckingham

Dying is a physical process; it is a psychological process; it is a spiritual and a social process. The process of dying is part of the process of living. We should not deny it. American perspectives on death and dying seem to be strangely paradoxical. Our news media confront the fact of death directly with statements that range from magnificent headlines to unobtrusive notices on the obituary page. On the other hand, we Americans generally prefer to speak about particular deaths rather than death in the abstract. In our culture speaking about death and dying has been a taboo topic. It has been taboo because it has been hidden. We Americans are continually hesitant to talk openly about the process of dying itself. We see this fact often demonstrated by the physician who hesitates to be totally honest with a patient. Physicians in this culture are trained to cure. When cure becomes impossible, the typical physician's response is to leave the patient alone and report to the family that all that medical science can do has been done. One must understand that physicians, like the rest of us, are trained and tempted by success. Death to them represents a failure, and failures are difficult to swallow.

In medical schools and hospitals, physicians and nurses may exhibit considerable skill in handling the medical mechanics of attending the dying. But rarely do they address the patient as a total person. Physicians and nurses also have trouble in dealing with the dying. After spending three years working as a researcher with terminal cancer patients, I have found that what these people need and want most is basic relief from the dignity-degrading symptoms of their disease, continuous competent medical care, and assurance that they won't be abandoned by the medical/nursing staff and their own loved ones.

"Hospice" is a medieval term denoting a place designed for the provision of comfort and hospitality to travelers along the road. For the American hospice, the road is the course of terminal illness, and the travelers are the patients whose prognosis precludes an aggressive rehabilitative endeavor. The New Haven-area hospice (with which I am most familiar) offers a kind of continuing health care that enables patients and families to live out their lives together as fully and comfortably as possible. Such care includes meeting the spiritual and emotional, as well as the medical, needs of the patient.

Hospice New Haven started a home care service for patients and their families in 1974. This service, tailored to meet the individual requirements of each patient, is administered by the full-time hospice physician and staffed by a team capable of fulfilling a broad spectrum of patient-family needs. The team consists of an additional physician, registered nurses, licensed practical nurses, a social worker, a researcher, a clinical pharmacist, clergy, other professionals as needed, and volunteers. By using such a blend of complementary professional, nonprofessional, and volunteer skills, the staff at the hospice developed a comprehensive, integrated, and complete care program, capable of specialized and consistent support of the patient and his family. Optimal provision of care calls for coordinated, collaborative effort on the part of the hospice team, which responds to the individual and diverse needs of the terminal patient.

By employing specialized, intensive medical, nursing, and pharmaceutical services, the treatment program is directed at controlling pain, nausea, and other correlates of terminal disease that deprive the patient of the strength needed to participate in living. Such symptom management enhances the quality of life by eliminating preoccupation with suffering and enabling the patient to remain comfortable, alert, and in good spirits during his last days. Hospice personnel, witnesses to disruption of the family life style by multiple changes that occur during terminal illness, recognize the importance of sustaining continuity of care. Because terminal illness upsets the equilibrium of the family group, it is the patient-family that is designated as the unit for care. Medical care and supportive counseling involve both the patient and family by day in their homes. The team is also on call for emergencies at night and on weekends. A vital aspect in maintaining family cohesion is the training of a "primary care person" in nursing methods, enabling active participation in and valuable contribution to the care of the patient. In addition, volunteers free more time for the family to draw closer to the patient and to themselves. By thus incorporating the family into the patient care system, the anguish of loneliness and isolation experienced by the patient is reduced, and the ability of the hospice team to provide support for the family before, during, and after the patient's death is greatly enhanced.

The goals of the hospice care program are:

a) to aid in reducing the burden of a traumatic life experience by sharing and meeting the expressed needs (physical, emotional, spiritual, and social) of the cancer patient and family;
b) to assist the patient to achieve and maintain maximum independent living and living with dignity until death;
c) to minimize the painful and damaging effects of the death of a family member upon the remaining family members.

Hospice projected a unique 44-bed facility to complete the total program. This facility was designed to supply inpatient care without the limitations of the acute-care hospital (e.g., visiting restrictions and aggressive therapy) and will especially aid the following:

— patients who, with additional support, could remain at home;
— people who are unable to cope any longer in their own homes;
— patients whose symptoms can be alleviated by round-the-clock attention;
— those whose families, wearied by prolonged nursing, need a rest themselves;
— those whose families have been unable to take a vacation because of their nursing commitment.

In endeavoring to provide the best possible terminal care to patients and their families, and in seeking to maximize opportunities for health care personnel to learn from close contact with the dying and the bereaved, the hospice is modeled after its British prototype, St. Christopher's, which was built in London in 1967. The hospice philosophy, both in London and in New Haven, emphasizes optimal use and flexibility of resources in caring for the patient and family. Basic to the hospice home care system is belief in the right of the terminal patient to die at home rather than in the depersonalizing surroundings of an acute-care hospital or nursing home.

By integrating humanistic medical and nursing care, hospice home care attempts to provide a warm atmosphere of peace and friendliness in which the patient can ask questions about his condition. Hospice is concerned with teaching health professionals and relatives of dying patients that evasion and deception only exacerbate the patient's difficulty in coping with illness. It is essential that both the staff and the patient be prepared to confront the whole truth about the imminence of death and that the staff be ready to listen supportively to the patient as the final stages of life and illness are resolved.

Maintenance of the family as a cohesive, supportive unit; provision for the relief of loneliness and separation anxiety; and symptom control for the maximum comfort and alertness of the dying patient are key objectives of the hospice staff in ensuring accessibility of professional and ancillary staff skills and in making arrangements for optimum care in a home environment.

If the needs of the family of the patient are inadequately attended to, attempts at meaningful care of the patient may be in vain. Thus, orientation toward both patient and family is a basic tenet of the hospice endeavor, and consideration of the family, often reluctant to disclose its own needs, is accepted as an essential component of home care. Only when feelings of anger, guilt, and loneliness experienced by the family members are vented and dissipated can the unspoken sense of alienation in the dying patient be alleviated. Family problems are often too closely related to interaction with the terminally ill cancer patient to go unheeded.

Patients' behavioral patterns often undergo a marked change, and overlapping defenses of denial and symptoms of depression dominate their relationships with others. At this time the medical team personnel, and more especially the families, desperately need to understand that the patients' changed behavior is a predictable response to a very difficult situation.

Even in its incipient stages, the comprehensive hospice home care program was seen as valuable insofar as it attained its goal of maintaining a quality of life satisfactory to both patient and family during that life's final stretch. Craven and Wald (1975) have stated that "what people need most when they are dying is relief from the distressing symptoms of their disease, the security of a caring environment, sustained expert care, and the assurance they and their families won't be abandoned" by family and caregivers. It is hoped that by eliminating the deficiencies in existing forms of terminal care, the hospice can meet such primary needs.

The Problem of Pain

The hospice program has evolved in part as an attempt to compensate for the inadequacies of the present medical system, acute-care hospitals, and physicians in relieving the physical distress of the terminal cancer patient. At present, we can only hope that the average terminal patient suffering from pain will find complete relief. Analgesic dosages are generally standardized and seldom calibrated to meet the patient's individual needs. Anxiety is provoked by anticipation of the cyclic return of pain, the inevitable consequence of inappropriate administration of drugs. Scheduling and apportioning of pain-relieving medications are seldom suited to the patient's requirements: the patient is often sentenced to pass through consecutive stages of sedation, uneasiness, and intense suffering. Narcotics prescribed to be given when needed are often withheld by members of the medical staff to avoid addiction; they are seldom administered before the patient is in a state of acute distress. The results can be inadequate relief of pain and decreasing potential for the realization of projected goals of pain control (Janzen 1974).

The majority of physicians who care for the terminally ill harbor fears of addiction, tolerance, and mental impairment in their patients and consequently prescribe narcotics on a four-hourly p.r.n. (pro re nata) or "as needed/when necessary" basis. Under this system of narcotic administration the patient must be in pain before he is able to receive the drug; if his therapeutic regimen calls for pain killer every four hours and he demonstrates a need for pain-relieving medication before that time has elapsed, he is left to suffer out the remaining interval in pain. The practice at St. Christopher's, in contrast, is to titrate the level of analgesic against the degree of pain experienced by the patient, increasing the dosage gradually until the pain is alleviated. The subsequent dose is given before the effects of the previous dose have subsided, and thus pain is kept in abeyance (Twycross 1974).

According to Mount (1976), there are several aims in treating the intractable pain of advanced cancer. Clarification of the cause of the pain is an essential first aim in symptom control and may suggest possible modes of therapeutic intervention. Awareness of the cause of the pain and the existence of effective therapies for its relief serve to remove the patient from the characteristic state of meaningless, helplessness, and hopelessness described by LeShan (1974). A second important aim is the anticipation and prevention of pain, as opposed to treatment of pain once it has occurred. As the anxious anticipation and memory of pain are lessened by repeated success at preventing pain, the amount of analgesic required for the maintenance of comfort frequently decreases (Mount 1976).

Another aim of the treatment of pain is achieving a pain-free state without sedation. Many patients feel that the only alternatives open to them are constant pain on the one hand and perpetual somnolence on the other. Comfort and an unclouded sensorium can be achieved simultaneously, however, if careful individual regulation of analgesic dosage is provided (Mount 1976). The ability to relate to his environment in a normal manner, neither euphoric due to an excess of drugs nor distressed due to inadequate medication, is a vital patient need. Even the mode of administration should be considered with the maximum benefit to the patient in mind: oral analgesia provides the patient with a degree of mobility and independence that is not afforded by parenteral administration (Mount 1976).

There is convincing evidence that the Brompton narcotic mixture, an oral narcotic preparation given with a phenothiazine, is an effective method for the control of severe pain. The mixture is used when milder narcotic and nonnarcotic preparations prove ineffective; yet, in spite of its potent analgesic effects, an anticipated protracted survival period is not a contraindication (Melzack 1973). With careful monitoring of the patient's needs and adjustment of dosage, the mixture may be used for many months and even several years without dose escalation.

In addition to the problem of pain, levels of anxiety and depression have been documented as the next most important variables to consider in rendering effective terminal care to patients and their families.

In a recently completed controlled study in which 38 hospice patients and primary care persons were matched in sex, primary site, and age, I have found the following enlightening and encouraging results in the hospice patients in comparison with the nonhospice group:

a) lower levels of anxiety and depression as measured by the Zuckerman and Lubin and Sympton Checklist 90 Scales,
b) higher levels of social adjustment as measured by the Social Adjustment Self-Report Questionnaire,
c) lower levels of anxiety and depression as measured by the Zuckerman and Lubin and Sympton Checklist 90 Scales,
d) higher levels of social adjustment as measured by the Social Adjustment Self-Report Questionnaire.

These findings were found statistically significant at the .01 level.

Primary care persons of both hospice and non-hospice origin experienced more friction with people around them than patients did from the respective study groups. Primary care persons were also, in general, more hostile and less anxious and depressed than patients. More significant differences were observed among primary care persons than among patients; hence, hospice services had a greater effect on primary care persons than on patients.

The emphasis of the hospice home care program is on the patient and family as the unit of care. Without a multidisciplinary team concept, the New Haven hospice home care program could not have succeeded.

In conclusion, I would like to state that I have some serious reservations about the future of hospice in America. Many developing hospice organizations throughout this country have become misdirected by what I call the "edifice complex," the major goal being the erection of a fancy structure—a temple to the dying. This edifice complex must be cured. We do not need more acute- or chronic-care beds in this country. We need to use the existing facilities we have. We need to emphasize the importance of home care for the dying. We need to direct our care to the patient and family as the unit of care.

We who care for the dying and their families must be willing to learn from our dying patients. In day-to-day life, it is easy for us to get wrapped up in the trivial concerns of existence. It is through the eyes of the dying that we can really see and appreciate the meaning and beauty of life.

References

Craven, J. and F. Wald. 1975. "Hospice Care for Dying Patients." *American Journal of Nursing* (October).

Janzen, E. 1974. "Relief of Pain." *Nursing Forum* 13:1.

Le Shan, L. 1974. "The World of the Patient in Severe Pain of Long Duration." *Journal of Chronic Disease* 17:119.

Melzack, R. 1973. *The Puzzle of Pain*. Harmondsworth, England: Penguin.

Mount, B. M. 1976. "Use of the Brompton Mixture in Treating the Chronic Pain of Malignant Disease." *Canadian Medical Association Journal* (July 17) 115:122-24.

Twycross, R. G. 1974. "Clinical Experience with Diamorphine in Advanced Malignant Disease." *International Journal of Clinical Pharmacology, Therapy, and Toxicology* 9:3.

31

Problems of Terminal Care: Behavioral Approaches and Environmental Stimulation

William Regelson and Brian West

While society gives the physician an important place in the care of the catastrophically ill (the preterminal), in reality our role is minimal except as a force for humanistic interaction (Regelson 1979, 1980, 1981). Any emphasis on the treatment of the catastrophically ill requires supportive care as its main prop, and medical measures can, to a large degree, be surrogated to paramedics, that is, nurse practitioners and physician's helpers, or to nurses, practical nurses, or family. More importantly, we must be aware of the important role behavioral psychologists can play as part of a supportive therapeutic team.

In any extended-care facility for the catastrophically or chronically ill that includes the home as a key factor in the supportive program, the major question governing the home environment is the capacity for self-help in the patient or the family. Typically, this relates to the degree of physical ability required to maintain toilet function, feeding capacity, and relief of pain and fear of abandonment.

When a patient can feed or wash himself, get to the toilet, or provide a positive interaction with those who support him, every effort should be made to keep that individual out of the hospital. A patient who requires a bedpan and hand feeding and lacks the ability to communicate or enjoy life can be sustained only when there is a pattern of social obligation based on love or guilt, or there is income support for home care to be made possible. The burden of care for any individual at home can be accommodated depending upon the degree of shared responsibility, economic costs, or income and the length of time that those responsible must sacrifice their personal and normal needs for the seriously ill.

The family's role is critical, and families vary in their capacity to provide nursing care. Home nursing is a socioeconomic problem, for tolerance to the patient is inversely proportional to hope for recovery and/or finances. The family's capacity to cope is related to the degree of the patient's self-help, but with increasing dependency, supportive systems have to be concerned with the length of time it takes for recovery or for relief to be afforded by the death of the patient. It is obvious that the length of an illness and its economic cost, as well as toilet or feeding needs that disturb the sleep, recreation, or work habits of the family, will seriously limit their capacity to cope in helping the patient.

All families involved in nursing at home care have their breaking point! In its minor manifestation, we have seen emergency room dumping where the family surrenders a relative over the weekend for the simple need to remove a fecal impaction or provide an enema. A minor problem can provide the family with the opportunity to take its vacation at the expense of abandoning their family responsibility to the patient for the vagaries of an emergency room. How many of us, as physicians, are induced to admit patients to hospitals with the cost paid by Medicare because a family cannot cope?

While caring for the catastrophically ill or helpless patient may be economically or socially equivalent to the cost of raising a child, it is obvious that there is no equivalent reward or emotional satisfaction for the same tasks. Here, we are faced with distinct social problems based on sex differences in those responsible for nursing. Women, in our society, are much better equipped to cope with the chronically ill because of social conditioning related to the woman's maternal role or her social preparation for housekeeping skills. One can chauvinistically relate this to intrinsic qualities in sex differences that we romanticize as being basic to a woman's role biologically. However, regardless of the intrinsic cause, it has been quite evident that men rarely play a supporting role of significance for the chronically ill unless there is a woman to help bear the burden. This is particularly true when illness will result in death.

Death and debility are frequently destructive to the participant or family who must sustain the victim unless measures are developed to maintain morale for both the patient and those involved in nursing. The role of guilt or the "common decency response" ("If I don't do it, who will?") is a factor in nursing the terminally ill, and often the spur to participation. This usually falls on one or two female family members, depending upon the size and structure of the family.

It must be remembered that guilt or the lack of shared responsibility fosters resentment, and resentment does not lead to good nursing care or to healthy family relationships before or after the death of the patient. It is for this reason that home care for the preterminal must not be an interminable burden for the family member doing the job or harboring the individual. It must be a shared responsibility requiring other family members and/or distinct professional support. It is mandatory that there be an opportunity for escape for the major person responsible for nursing within a family home circumstance.

In our experience, one of the major problems of home care, particularly for the elderly, is the total destruction of normal sleep patterns because of the patient, who frequently cannot tell day from night. Physical consequences of the absence of sleep can be totally destructive to morale and physical capacity to cope with even simple tasks. One cannot expect good nursing supportive care from a family member if the sleep pattern is destroyed because of the needs of the patient. For this reason, one of the major roles of the physician is to provide hypnotic or sedative relief for the patient in an effort to restore normal sleep patterns. Unfortunately, as there is no really good drug for us, frequently a drugged, oftentimes confused, continually sedated patient is, in effect, suffering premature death by having his faculties limited by the need to provide sleep.

While the need for sleep is most often the patient's, it is the supportive family member who also must have a decent night's sleep to continue to cope with the patient or the demands of a job or of maintaining the family. This is one major reason why institutional care can be more effective than home care. One of the major priorities of medicine should be to develop drugs or techniques (e.g., electrically induced sleep) that can induce regular patterns of sleep for the patient without clouding sensibility or producing narcotic dependency. Thus, normal patterns of interaction to meet the needs of those who have to interface with the patient on a daily basis can be supported. Characteristically, there is always one member of the family who bears the burden as a result of many factors, ranging from availability to love, to geography, to guilt, to hopes of reward in the patient's will. Those responsible for home care must protect the nursing family member lest the opportunities and length of time available for the patient in the home environment be limited. For this reason, there must be trained workers with knowledge of the family structure and the sociology of the particular ethnic groups involved who can adjudicate care burdens in advance of the crisis leading to the patient's debility and death. Above all, there must be an opportunity for transfer of the patient from the home to a hospice structure for nonmedical, social, and nursing reasons to relieve an overburdened family member who is being destroyed by the nursing role.

Many hospitals do provide counseling, psychotherapy, chaplain services, and social worker services that not only respond to current psychosocial problems but also anticipate them. An example of this is the rehabilitation and continuing care project for cancer patients, now in progress in our own institution (Medical College of Virginia), that utilizes a team or multidisciplinary treatment approach. We feel that a thorough knowledge and understanding of the patient's problems must necessarily precede or be an integral part of treatment programs. In regard to the physician's responsibility, our experience has shown that supportive drug therapy is only one part of a cancer patient's needs.

Past experiences with multidisciplinary approaches to the social and psychologic impact of medical problems have been important to the overall treatment of the patient (Lewis 1978). Evidence supports the fact that primary care is benefited by means of adjunctive psychological and sociological treatment that facilitates more rapid or complete physical recovery. It is important to begin such treatment before problems develop rather than to act when life stress, that is, physical, social, and economic problems, creates crises.

One reason for the absence of the universal application of holistic-multidisciplinary teams concerned with psychosocial factors in primary care is the absence of applied validity measures. Hospital administrators and physicians cannot judge the cost-effectiveness of any treatment by subjective opinions. The worth of a systematic assessment of any procedure is the ability to establish goals and obtain quantifiable results; it is increasingly important to ask if a program will shorten the time the patient is confined to the hospital bed. If a program accelerates a patient's return to home and to an improved participation in life or as a contributing economic member of the community, one must ask if this approach to patient care provides a positive change in the quality of life the patient experiences.

To carry out our program, we developed a therapeutic team with an élan and identity of its own that was well integrated with preexisting procedures and personnel. (Unfortunately, it no longer exists, because the program was not funded.) Such a team should be economically integrated and include psychiatrists, psychologists, psychiatric nurses, social workers, rehabilitation counselors, physical therapists, and a variety of paraprofessionals in addition to the primary physician. This emphasis on a multidisciplinary group permits an integration of health care with a more global view of the patient's needs. An informational approach to patient support or therapy provides the background for a program in "holistic care" that can take place in any setting—home, hospital, or hospice.

The following is a statement and a summary of what we feel is necessary for the care of the terminally ill.

A. Holistic Approach to Patient Care:
   1. This approach reflects the philosophy that hospitals and hospital staff can no longer be responsible only for patients' physical well-being, but also must be responsible for providing services that will aid the patient in other aspects of life that may be affected by the disease.

   It must be stressed that supportive therapy cannot be confined to drugs alone. As defined under the heading of "Holistic Medicine," psychosocial measures are necessary adjuncts equal to supportive drugs in surgery, to radiotherapy and to chemotherapy as these are given to cancer patients. In our work, we attempted to develop a team concept of patient evaluation and support that made visible the economic and social benefits gained in providing for the total needs of patients with catastrophic disease—the relief of symptoms, the shortening of hospital time, and the rehabilitation of patients for more effective survival.

It has been our experience, in a three-year program, that a supportive team primarily concerned with the evaluation of drug responses was a partially wasted resource unless it also concerned itself with psychosocial factors, supportive counseling, and the patient's environment.

B. The "Kinesthetic Room" and the "Living Window":

The existing stimulation provided for patients in most hospitals or nursing home situations consists of a television set, a radio, and a window. Even with cable television and new cassette opportunities, the availability of appropriate programs for patient stimulation is frequently limited. What we were seeking to create was a "kinesthetic room" and/or "living window" that could be tailor-made to suit the needs of individual patients, or patients in selected disease categories, faced with sensory deprivation because of chronic illness or confinement. This technology of controlled environmental stimulation has been applied to crewmen on atomic submarines, and there is an absolute need to extend it as an option to other sensory deprived members of our society.

The technology we employed consisted of the following:

1. "The Living Window": This used pictures of flowers, trees, familiar scenes, and exotic imagery presented by color slide projection and film technology.

Key features of this type of programming were:

(a) Use of pictures of loved ones, episodes of past and present (pictures of early life, marriage, birthdays, weddings, trips) that could be included in the pictorial representation from the patient's own experience (photograph collections). We called this "The Time Machine."

(b) Use of "retroscreen technology" or its equivalent (hydraulic head camera mounts for filming family photographs or magazine illustrations) to utilize still films to provide moving imagery of striking emotional impact. For example, we can fixate on the pupil of the eye, which can then be expanded into the entire eye, the face, and then the full figure in a specific setting. One can look at the center of the flower, then the full flower, and finally the field in which it grows.

(c) The development of archetypal imagery as a therapeutic tool to help patients cope with disease. Visual imagery can help patients' attitudes toward procedures, that is, minor surgery, pain, etc. Pictorial sources for this work can be obtained from magazines or film collections.

2. The "Living Window" sequence was enhanced by music accompaniment to the changing images. The taste of the individual relevant to classical, country, jazz or pop music was a critical consideration as was concern for the mood change to be produced or reinforced. (We used a "Chinese Menu" to aid in film and music sequencing. "Select from column A or column B.")

This type of kinesthetic sensation using changing perspectives (zoom) in still pictures had an aesthetic appeal in producing mood effects quite different from ones created with ordinary motion picture technology. This is particularly true when combined with music. Further development associated with this should be carried out.

3. The "Kinesthetic Technologist": The development of programs to require the training of a new technologist was begun in conjunction with the art and music and psychology departments of Virginia Commonwealth University (V.C.U.). It is still under development, that is, to train a professional person similar to those individuals, for example, engaged in "art or music therapy." These people will, based upon experience and training, develop programs for individuals and for whole groups within particular disease categories. They will establish and govern the administration of programs in cooperation with physicians, psychologists, and family.

4. "Olfactory Stimulation": We had a chemical engineer who was developing a program to give us up to 14 different odors, for example, roasting coffee, pine scent, chocolate, flowers. A button push will provide olfactory stimulation that is readily changed to meet or modify moods. Olfaction provides a "Proustian option" that can strikingly affect memory, feelings, and attitudes of the individual patient who is confined to the kinesthetic room.

5. "Sun Wall": We hoped to have special lighting techniques that could imitate the sun migrating across the sky and provide morning shadows, midday overhead light, or afternoon shadows that again change the character of mood.

6. "Feel Texture": We also planned to use the opportunity to stimulate

touch. We developed plans for a mobile that could be lowered from the ceiling to provide the individual with various textures: satin, silk, velour, marble, etc., so that childlike primitive feeling related to feeling texture could be introduced.

7. "Touch Stimulation": In addition, and more important to this program, we would seek to restore the *back rub* and *massage* as a therapeutic factor. Being touched, to produce pleasure, could be a critical feature of this program. Nurses no longer do this, but it was to be part of the opportunities provided for patients in the kinesthetic setting.

Discussion:

The preliminary experience with the "Kinesthetic Room" and "Living Window" showed that it could provide alternatives for the growing number of patients suffering from chronic disease and debility. As our population ages, chronic illness becomes a serious social problem. Prolonged hospitalization or confinement to a bedroom or nursing home often result. Studies in our cancer patient population, which served us in this study, are broadly applicable to the wide range of patients chronically ill and debilitated.

Confinement, that is, the inability to change one's environment through one's own direct efforts, has many depressive side effects. Sensory deprivation, the boredom and despair that are associated with being in restricted, limited environments (the single room or the institutional environment of a nursing home or hospital) must be altered to provide options for controlled stimulation.

Our program showed that through visual images and music, mood and attitude can be altered to provide alternatives to boredom, hopelessness, and anxiety in cancer patients. If these programs can achieve proper support, it will eventually provide for the development of a professionally trained technologist who will put together individual programs for patient needs, as well as alternative methods of stimulation, including odor, light (control of shadows), and touch (including the restoration of massage). We predict that environmental stimulation and conditioning can provide for a new world of therapy for the cancer patient and should be supported by the National Institutes of Health and hospices.

C. Alternative Approaches Other than Supportive Drugs or the Kinesthetic Room:

While the primary emphasis of our program was on the evaluation of supportive drugs, as part of our program we developed a supportive therapy team into a structure for the holistic care and evaluation of patients.

The following is intended as a brief introduction to some of the techniques that have been investigated and used successfully in many clinical situations (Rimm and Masters 1974) and that we started to use. These techniques were intended for problem-oriented, short-term therapy.

1. Biofeedback

Biofeedback is the term applied to a system for providing to an organism information about ongoing biological activity. The result is self-control of some types of physiological activity, particularly those related to psychological stress. Sensory mechanisms (i.e., electrodes) detect the activity (i.e., muscle tension), and this information, or signal, is amplified into a visual or auditory feedback display (Brown 1977). Biofeedback can be especially helpful for patients, enabling them to learn to depend more on internal control than on the therapists or pharmacological agents (Brown 1977).

Other modalities of biofeedback have also been successfully used. For example, measuring blood pulse volume in the temporal artery of migraine headache patients, Koppman et al. (1974) reported less pain (subjective) and a reduction in the frequency of their patient's headaches.

2. Contingency Management (Contracting)

Based on the idea that our actions are under the control of rewards and punishments that we receive in our environment, contracting systematically manipulates situations and the consequent reward and punishment in order to change behavior. Persons benefiting from this treatment are those who indulge in self-defeating behaviors owing to the deficiency of immediate or potential rewards available in the environment, especially those that elicit more appropriate behavior. Problems such as overeating or undereating, excessive drinking or smoking, lack of exercise, and inability to maintain strict medication schedules can be successfully treated with contingency management. The reward system can consist of pleasant or positive effects elicited by supportive drugs or an opportunity to participate in the environment of the "kinesthetic room."

3. Progressive Muscle Relaxation

Approaching a state of muscle relaxation, a person's tension and anxiety are drastically reduced. This procedure involves a series of "exercises" of successive tensing and relaxing major muscle groups so that a state of muscle relaxation may be attained. It can be used together with biofeedback for training purposes.

4. Systematic Desensitization

This treatment utilizes muscle relaxation, cognitive imagery tapes, and TV imagery (i.e., the kinesthetic room) to reduce anxiety and fear (i.e., phobias) of particular situations or objects. Phobias develop through anxiety reactions to particular situations. These reactions may become so severe that the person will avoid these situations. Many phobias or situationally specific fears can be disruptive to a person's everyday life, or even to his medical treatment. Excessive fear of medical surroundings or particular procedures may be treated by using systematic desensitization, and medical treatment and recovery may thus be facilitated.

The kinesthetic room showed that it could provide distraction from painful procedures (venipuncture). Delta-9-THC, the active ingredient of marijuana, was a useful psychoactive agent for this procedure.

5. Cognitive Approaches

An individual's thoughts and beliefs affect the way he feels and acts. Cognitive methods attempt to change behavior and emotion by dealing directly with beliefs and thought processes.

Rational emotive therapy assumes that psychological disorders are the result of faulty or irrational beliefs. When a person is exposed to an external event, thoughts and self-verbalizations result. Emotional reactions and behaviors are a result of these thoughts, and it is the therapist's job to help the patient examine and modify these thoughts.

In summary, programs for terminal care or catastrophic disease that are based on home or hospice care should have the following:

1. Programming to aid family members or friends participating in nursing by providing rotational voluntary or professional relief.
2. Convenient opportunities for transfer of patients to hospital or hospice institutions from the home for justified social as well as medical reasons.
3. Holistic care programs that include:

   (a) kinesthetic room; living window (controlled environments provide visual, auditory, and olfactory stimuli to allow the patient to escape from boredom and sensory deprivation).

   (b) Individuals trained in communication techniques and rehabilitation procedures who can make film and music presentations for the specific needs of patients.

   (c) Psychological behavioral programs in:

   (1) Biofeedback

   (2) Contingency management

   (3) Progressive muscle relaxation

   (4) Systematic desensitization and

   (5) Cognitive approaches

Biofeedback has a particularly successful place in relieving pain and anxiety. *Behavioral psychologists must be part of the supportive team dealing with the patient and the family to conduct these programs.*

4. Physicians and pharmacologists to develop more effective hypnotics and antiemetics for clinical needs.
5. Physical therapy, including back rubs and massage, to provide pleasure and anticipatory support for the terminally ill.
6. More emphasis on the development of attitudinal interactions and supportive environments in conjunction with drugs or placebo use to more effectively reinforce the positive action of drugs in relation to patient's needs. We have a difficult therapeutic problem in terminal patients when supportive drugs frequently prove inadequate or produce complicating side effects. In evaluating drug action, one must also decide between the obliterative effects of drugs on human personality and the comfort of the patient. In addition to therapy and analgesics or psychoactives, supporting medical personnel and family must be made aware that the dying cancer patient must have something to look forward to other than the grave, even if life is limited to days or weeks. It is our experience that drugs alone do not suffice for adequate control of the preterminal patient's symptoms. Placebo responses are valid, and the therapeutic conditioning role of the medical staff must be backed by a strong belief system in the value of their physical presence and the effectiveness of their drugs.
7. Evaluation systems to determine the success of such programs to justify their cost.

It should be the goal of supportive programs for the terminally ill to give patients something to look forward to in their day-to-day experience, no matter how limited. We must provide appropriate drugs, psychotherapy, physical therapy, massage, and supportive environments to correct or positively alter the cognitive and/or behavioral attitudes of the seriously ill that are detrimental to the quality of survival.

References

Brown, B. B. 1977. *Stress and the Art of Biofeedback*. New York: Harper and Row.

Regelson, W. 1979. "Aphorisms for Catastrophic Illness." *Resident and Staff Physician* 25:45-47.

———— 1980. *Medical Times* 108:89-93.

Regelson, W. 1980. "The Physician's Role in Catastrophic Disease." In P. Tretter et al., *Psychosocial Aspects of Radiation Therapy: The Patient, the Family, and the Staff,* New York: Arno Press.

Rimm, D. C. and J. C. Masters. 1974. *Behavior Therapy: Techniques and Empirical Findings*. New York: Academic Press.

Part VII

A Look to the Future

32

Health in the 1980s: Toward Optimum Human Existence

Russell Jaffe

Our view and definition of health determine our research and clinical strategies. At this time, limited research funding and clinical expenditures encourage the clearest and most productive definition of health.

Since the founding of our nation, the process of reexamining the fundamental framework of how we view and define health has roughly followed a 30-year cycle. The reexaminations have characteristically been generated by small, less orthodox groups within the medical community. Together with consumers, these groups, in spite of resistance from the prevailing health lobbies, have been able to initiate changes that have expanded the scope and use of health care professionals and benefited the community in general. The issues that usually stimulate change in health care are:

Option 1. insufficient scientific and technological bases for our medical and health strategies; or
Option 2. insufficient relevant personal and community health services.

In addition, when viewed from a broad perspective (200 plus years), we discern a pendulum moving from option 1 to option 2 and back.

At present, we find ourselves poised at the extreme of one expression of option 1 (more technology); yet a rising voice is heard for option 2 (more emphasis on personal and environmental health). Those who are developing new approaches to health are implicitly operating from an option 2 premise. In essence, we are at (or are just returning from) the extreme of one swing of the pendulum; the return of the pendulum may well characterize new approaches to health for the 1980s.

The middle of the nineteenth century saw an illuminating comparison of these issues in the form of the debate between Louis Pasteur and August Beauchamp. Pasteur focused his attention on external causes (infectious agents, environmental toxins, dietary problems, and natural allergens) as the primary threats to health. Beauchamp, on the other hand, viewed internal factors (the body's natural defense and immune system; the neuroendocrine system, especially the thyroid, thymus, and adrenal glands; fatigue, and the emotional and intellectual orientation of the person) as primary causes in susceptibility or resistance to health threats. Essentially, proponents of Pasteur hold that molecular biology research and technology can improve personal health quality, while those in support of Beauchamp believe that life-style and personal attitudinal integrity are the primary determinants of personal health quality. The most recent historic 30-year cycle, which chronologically has ended, has been overwhelmingly dominated by the Pasteurian view.

The Pasteurians tend to hold that objective scientific facts will lead the way to the eradication of disease; the Beauchampists favor a reliance on subjective experience as the more direct route to avoiding disease. This debate began during the mid-nineteenth century when Pasteur and Beauchamp each led medical research institutes in France.

The approach of Pasteur dominated overwhelmingly during the 1950s and 1960s. Within the past decade the debate has again become heated and enlivened. At present, we stand poised for new work in health. A consensus conceptualization of what some of this work may contain is my focal point here.

New work in health usually arises to meet some perceived need. Among today's perceived needs are:

a) slowing the escalation of health costs (which rise twice as fast as the GNP as a whole);

b) reducing chronic illness among teenagers (which doubled in the last decade);

c) rediscovering the primary importance of fulfilling human relationships and their role in health;

d) developing strategies to attain optimum human health and reduce our biosocial decline;

e) working toward voluntary and conscious control of automatic function;

f) exploring fields of contemplation, meditation, and spiritual inspiration in relation to attaining and maintaining health;

g) investigating genetic engineering to produce complex biological products such as the proteins, insulin, growth hormone, and interferon (which specially produced bacteria were first induced to synthesize during 1979);

h) investigating the role of laughter in attaining and maintaining health;

i) emphasizing the importance of self-care in health;

j) learning to recognize subtle signals given by the body when it is in a state of balance or unbalance with distress or disease (thus rediscovering that the human body is its own laboratory);

k) exploring the roles of the electromagnetic field in health, medical diagnosis, medical treatment, and health optimization;

l) investigating the biochemical, environmental, and social causes for ecologic sensitivity (such as food "allergy") and "executive fatigue syndrome";

m) studying the impact of environmental lighting, air, electricity, sound, water, quality, and synthetic materials on the body's natural defenses and the manner in which these factors predispose people to be susceptible to or resist illness;

n) extending our concepts of human growth and development to their broadest demonstrable limit; and

o) investigating, in a respectful manner, other cultures and the use of efficacious approaches toward health maintenance and disease reduction.

In essence, we are examining the fundamental assumptions upon which our health and research strategies have been based for the last generation. We may have the extraordinary fortune to be participatory witnesses of a shift from a narrow view of health (which focuses primarily on disease treatment and prevention) toward a broad view defining health in terms of the positive quality in soil, water, atmosphere, energy, and industrial output and leading to healthy food, healthy environments, and healthy people.

We are reaping the fruits of an intensive and productive generation of molecular biology research in medicine. Ushered in by the Salk-Enders-Sabin polio vaccine (in the early 1950s), this work is bringing noninvasive analysis of blood flow to the heart (scinticardiography—the use of a radioisotope that the heart muscle extracts and concentrates from the blood. With the help of computers, real time image of the beating heart can be constructed and displayed.); monitoring of the heart beat and muscular tone of the infant before delivery (thereby alerting the doctor to "fetal distress" if it should occur); long-term total intravenous feeding of the chronically ill or seriously disabled person, and so forth.

Medical information doubles every five years. Among the most important results of our rapidly expanding body of scientific and medical knowledge is the recognition that much previous medical "fact" is now clearly seen as "fiction." For instance, our attention to dietary cholesterol as a significant risk factor in our epidemic rise of cardiovascular diseases is now known to be based on a misinterpretation of the facts. Indeed, except in a tiny fraction of people (less than 1/2 of 1 percent) who have a genetic inability to metabolize blood fat, there is no direct relationship between dietary cholesterol and blood cholesterol. Rather, we are coming to recognize that abnormal laboratory results—for instance, an elevated blood cholesterol—are a reflection of some imbalance in the body. When the cause of the imbalance is discerned and balance reestablished, the abnormal laboratory result usually normalizes on its own. On the other hand, when the imbalance is allowed to persist, medications are often ineffective. Until recently, this anomaly has been mysterious. Today, it is an exciting frontier in medicine.

Another myth now disproven is the concept that much chronic illness is genetic. (By chronic illness is meant arthritis, heart disease, arteriosclerosis, stroke, obesity, diabetes.) While it is still sometimes taught that these conditions "run in families" and are, therefore, genetic, an accumulating body of wisdom suggests that families perpetuate certain life-styles and environments that are more directly responsible for these diseases of modern civilization than the genetic material or DNA is. An extension of this concept is the recognition that these genetic disabilities should remit and disappear if the life-style or environmental conditions responsible for their persistence are removed.

Such is frequently the case. Atherosclerosis—a cardiovascular condition leading to hardened blood vessels—is now increasingly recognized as a reversible condition. If this were principally a genetic expression, reversibility would be most unlikely. The fact that reversal or regression of arteriosclerosis, arthritis, diabetes, and so forth, does occur in some cases is a favorable prognosis for the future of our health and that of our children if we implement the proper life-styles and healthy environments.

On the other hand, it is understandable that these chronic disabilities will continue to afflict increasing numbers of Americans—and all those who lead our typical environmental life-style—because most health professionals do not yet have the benefit of being taught what to do in light of the insight alluded to above. Specifically, we can expect more emphasis on healthy food, nutrition, air and water quality, attitudinal maturity, and self-responsibility for health as the biomedical research of the 1980s yields fruit.

Another frontier of biomedicine in the 1980s is the recognition that each of us is his/her own laboratory control. In other words, it is increasingly clear that comparing individuals to laboratory results obtained on a "similar" population is, at best, a deceptively crude approximation. This topic is explored experimentally by Dr. George Z. William, previously of the National Institutes of Health, and theoretically by the outstanding biostatistician, Dr. Alvan Feinstein of Yale. Both reach the same conclusion. In simplified form, their work argues that, just as our fingerprints and faces are unique, so is our metabolic personality. Hence, it is wise to profile us during health as a control for the future. Subsequently, we can be compared to our own prior control values to determine impending or present disability. Dr. William shows that this approach can yield premonitory evidence of illness—sometimes years before any gross symptoms appear. Obviously, the earlier an imbalance is detected, the easier is its remediation. What is now known for a few thousand fortunate Americans may become the standard of care for all of us in the near future.

New work in health includes psychology, psychiatry, and the emerging sciences of psychobiology and transpersonal humanistic psychology. As the last two terms imply, they represent syntheses and logical/experiential extensions of earlier conceptual frameworks—notably by Freud, Adler, Jung, Sullivan, and Rogers.

Psychobiology explores the functioning of mind through interactive tools of psychologic evaluation complemented by biochemistry. Perhaps the most notable example of this domain is the recognition that truly new learning and brain sprouting can take place in the fully mature and adult brain—given optimum conditions. Notable in this field is Gary Lynch, Ph.D., who shows that at high potassium concentrations, mature brain cells can develop new interconnections. The salt potassium is concentrated intracellularly. This is in contrast to sodium, which is generally excluded from cells and exists in high concentration in the circulatory system. Foods rich in potassium (and other nutrients) are traditionally viewed as "brain foods" in indigenous cultures. These "brain foods" include bananas, similar fruits, and fresh vegetable juices. We are just beginning to rediscover the importance of nutrition in lifelong learning. In a similar fashion, we are discovering that optimum learning occurs in an atmosphere of relaxed, comfortable informality. Remember what your classrooms were like? This approach, called superlearning or suggestology, derives from the Bulgarian Dr. George Lazanov and is being extended by innovative educators in the United States. Both learning disabled and gifted children (and adults) show accelerated learning curves and improved retention under these conditions. A similar approach known as neurolinguistic reprogramming—an extension of Eriksonian hypnosis with a liberal admixture of practical spirituality and suggestology—is a promising application to human growth and psychological maturation.

Bibliography

Benson, H. 1975. *The Relaxation Response*. New York: William Morrow.

Cousins, N. 1979. *Anatomy of An Illness*. New York: Norton.

Ferguson, T., ed. "Medical Self-Care." Inverness, California: Medical Self-Care Press.

Frank, J. 1973. *Persuasion and Healing*. Baltimore: The Johns Hopkins University Press.

Genetic Engineering in the 1980's. 1980. *The Wall Street Journal* (January 22) :1.

Leichtman, R. and C. Japikse. "Health and Its Attainment." Columbus, Ohio: Ariel Press.

Lerner, M. In press. *The Bio-Social Decline Hypothesis.*

Lynch, J. 1977. *The Broken Heart.* New York: Basic Books.

Moody, R. 1978. *Laugh After Laugh.* Jacksonville, Florida: Headwaters Press.

Robinson, V. 1929. *Path Finders in Medicine.* Medical Life Press.

Schwartz, J. 1979. *Voluntary Control.* New York: Dutton Paperbacks.

Knowles, J. 1977. "Spending More and Feeling Worse." *Daedalus* 106 (Winter): 57-80.

33

Relating Medicine to Education— A Curriculum Outline

Arlene Seguine

While contemporary science creates new measures of maturity known as prolongevity and scholars complement their achievements by formulating new definitions of life with fresh perceptions of dying, the average citizen often opts to abdicate his responsibility for providing personal care for the terminally ill relative and for making funeral arrangements for the deceased. Therefore, it is now essential that within the purview of thanatology we reassess the hospice concept within the American health care delivery system.

The time is opportune for a fresh point of view in discussions that presently seem to be obsessed with death. The two dominant yet opposing schools of thought are the pessimistic, with its emphasis on suppressing the ritualistic and humanistic facets of the dying process, and the optimistic, with its propensity for promising added seasons to the life cycle that may yet prove eternal. This does not preclude the current existential viewpoint that man is amorphous and socially impotent, a credo further emphasized by the nihilistic philosophy that promotes the notions of denial and despair in the contemplation of death.

While death has "come out of the closet," it behooves the optimistic philosophers to initiate a positive perspective. One of the most logical vehicles lies in the hospice program. The hospice network (National Hospice Organization 1980) existing throughout the United States provides the strongest potential collective influence to help bridge the credibility gap between the positive and negative thinkers already identified and to furnish communication for reestablishing death as a home-based event with professional medical support systems (Ward 1978).

Such an interface helps strengthen the lifeline between the patient and the family with respect to the psychosocial dynamics of the whole grief continuum. But it requires the cooperation of scholars in academia and practitioners in medicine. Death's mystique may still disclose hidden dimensions of life yet to be unraveled by gerontologists and biophilosophers. Since many universities are affiliated with hospitals or medical centers, it seems logical to design curricula addressing the medical and educational components common to training medical students and allied health educators involved in the death experience housed within a hospice program (including home care). Such an educational enterprise would serve as a prototype for embracing positive strategies to cope with death in a society imbued with tacit repudiations of the final rite of passage.

This particular course/curriculum should embody an interdisciplinary knowledge base that integrates the psychomotor, cognitive, and affective domains of learning. Within this spectrum would be learning experiences related to death education, psychology of dying, bioethics, counseling of dying patients, administration and organization of hospice programs, social gerontology, exercise modules, and so forth. Such a range of academic preparation equips the potential hospice professional with the breadth of expertise commensurate with the holistic concept of medical care currently being generated.

The framework for a curriculum that interfaces medicine with education is depicted by the flow chart (Fig. 33.1) included here. The schematic illustrates how different clusters of courses feed into one another. The trio of courses in the upper left-hand corner (sociology of medicine, medicolegal aspects of hospices, and pharmacopoeia of pain)

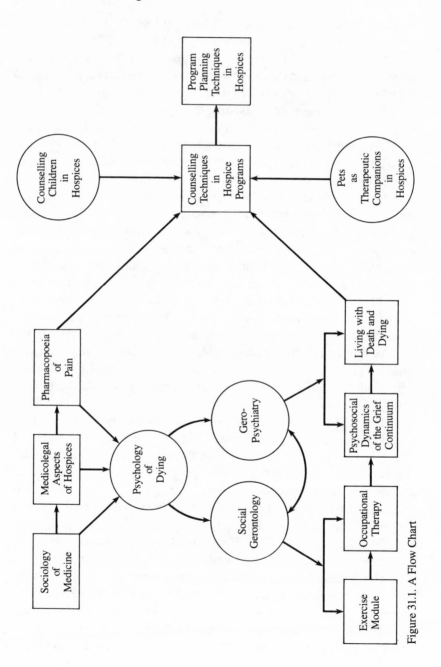

Figure 31.1. A Flow Chart

are in the cognitive domain of learning and relate to the sociobioethic dimensions of patient care. In addition, they form the foundation for flowing into the triad of courses (psychology of dying, social gerontology, and geropsychiatry) that integrates cognitive and affective components while providing for branching into the psychomotor domain included in exercise module and occupational therapy. The latter two are counterbalanced by the intersecting of the cognitive with the affective dimensions of psychosocial dynamics of the grief continuum and living with death and dying.

Together this constellation of courses, which covers the spectrum of cognitive, affective, and psychomotor facets of instruction, naturally combines and funnels into the counseling cluster.

Bibliography

Bibb, P. I. 1979. "Therapy for Intractable Pain." *Cancer Nursing* 2:247-48.

Bowers, M. K. et al. 1975. *Counseling the Dying*. New York: Jason Aronson, Inc.

Butler, R. N., and M. Lewis. 1977. *Aging and Mental Health*. St. Louis, Missouri: C. V. Mosby Company.

Davidson, G. W., ed. 1978. *The Hospice: Development and Administration*. Washington: Hemisphere Publishing Corporation.

Davis, H. J. 1978. "Brompton's Cocktail: Making Good-byes Possible." *American Journal of Nursing* 78:610-12.

Evans, C. 1979. "Hospice Program to Start." *New York Times* (December 30).

Garfield, C. 1978. *Psychosocial Care of the Dying Patient*. New York: McGraw Hill.

Kastenbaum, R. and R. Aisenberg. 1972. *The Psychology of Death*. New York: Springer Publishers.

Kron, J. 1979. "Designing a Better Place to Die." *New York Magazine* (March 1): 43-44.

Lamb, L. 1979. "Hospice U. S. A." *The Health Letter* (February): 1.

McMahon, J. and B. Woller-Lowrie. 1979. "Death and Dying: Hospice Programs." *Gannett Westchester Newspaper* (September 27): 11-13.

McMillan, N. P. 1980. "The Film Diary of a Terminal Care Patient." *New York Times* (January 20).

National Hospice Organization. 1980. *Directory of Hospices* (Tower Suite 506), 301 Maple Avenue, Vienna, Virginia, 22180.

Paige, R. L. and J. F. Looney. 1978. "Hospice Care for the Adult." In R. Fulton et al., *Death and Dying: Challenge and Change*. Reading, Massachusetts: Addison-Wesley.

Rossman, P. 1978. *Creating New Models of Care for the Terminally Ill*. Chicago: Association Press/Follett.

Ryder, C. F. and D. M. Ross. 1978. "Terminal Care: Issues and Alternatives." In R. Fulton, et al., *Death and Dying: Challenge and Change*. Reading, Massachusetts: Addison-Wesley.

Saunders, C. 1978. "Should a Patient Know?" In R. Fulton et al., *Death and Dying: Challenge and Change*. Reading, Massachusetts: Addison-Wesley.

Stoddard, S. 1978. *The Hospice Movement*. New York: Random House.

Sudnow, D. 1967. *Passing On: The Social Organization of Dying*. Englewood Cliffs, New Jersey: Prentice-Hall.

Ward, B. J. 1978. "Hospice Home Care Program." *Nursing Outlook* 26 (10):646-49.

Weisman, A. D. 1972. *On Dying and Denying: A Psychiatric Study of Terminality*. New York: Human Sciences Press.

34

Patient Support
in the 21st Century

Leonard M. Liegner and Ellen Martin

Join us on a time machine to the twenty-first century to take a look at continuing care *support* services (and please note the emphasis).

The medical care system experienced in the 1980s, as far as supportive patient care was concerned, was in a shambles. Scientific medicine dehumanized the patient, and its adherents incorrectly believed that they as providers did the patient a favor when, in fact, the patient was doing the provider a favor by permitting the physician and the staff to care for him. Health care providers were employed by the patient, a fact we now recognize in 2001. The patient had a right to discharge the physician unilaterally but rarely acted upon that right. If the patient had done so more often, we might have reached the present era sooner.

A dream! Attractive surroundings and magnificent trees and flowers. No resisting sitting on this bench by the fountain before entering what in the old days might have been called a hospital but now might be a "continuing care support center."

We remember Cecily Saunders, the hospice at St. Christopher's, and their global influence to focus care once again on patients as people.

We will never forget the warmth and devotion of her and her staff to the totality of spirit, mind, and body.

Twenty years have passed and what wonderful changes in medical care have occurred! Society has unreservedly committed more than adequate funds to the spiritual, emotional, environmental, and physical health of our citizens. The billions of dollars wasted on armaments have been redistributed to man's improvement rather than to his destruction. In this twenty-first century, love, peace, and understanding have been realized.

The revolution in interactional computer communications has brought us as *individuals* back into the picture. Before interactional computer systems, unilateral decisions were made by the establishment. Through the power of the ever-present moment-to-moment feedback, the present system evolved. Voting machines failed to do it; politicians made promises and failed to deliver. Now, with instant feedback opinion, no central authority can be the sole decision-maker for our own existence and survival. No politician, as we have seen in the last twenty years, can isolate himself behind the barrier of quotes. The change began with a recognition that information is secondary since it can be obtained basically from the portable microminicomputers that are carried with us. Students and teachers concentrate on human interrelationships in regular, ongoing emotional sensitivity training rather than on facts. There is no resemblance to the failing educational system of the 1980s. Psychotherapy is readily available for all and socially acceptable.

No longer are physicians the high-risk group for drug and alcohol abuse, divorce, and suicide. Medical schools are now multivaried. Those who wish to become caregiving doctors (in the olden days they might have been called bedside family doctors) are carefully selected, not by high grades in physics and laboratory chemistry but by the strength of their backgrounds in humanities, sociology, and psychology. Individual and group psychotherapy experiences, inconceivable in 1980, are mandatory for one year prior to entry into this branch of the medical health science center. Additionally, the candidate must have shown prior documented interest in an actual service facility. Those who wish to be doctors but who are not interested in direct people care form a different pool of students and could be considered more like the Ph.D.s in physics, chemistry, biochemistry, and physiology of the 1980s. They go along a different track and make their contributions in laboratories or in clinical research settings.

In the modern era, the caregiving physician is completely in charge of all medical matters and responsible to the patient directly. On all levels of care, the physician is employed *by the patient* in the full sense. The twenty-first-century caregiver/physician is aware of himself as a feeling human being before becoming a doctor. Individual and group psychosocial awareness training have assured the selection of a caring human being into the medical school.

Medical schools have now altered the dehumanizing influence of the previously isolating preclinical years and its concentration on a basic science by providing early patient contact for the medical student in the context of psychosocial orientation. As we remember, there was a doctor who was doing this at a major urban medical center during those past years. There were a few medical students then who were fortunate enough to have accepted that experience.

The ultimate goal of the health science center is the development of mature, caregiver physicians. In the continuing care support centers, we no longer have psychosocially ignorant physicians or those with overblown egos who cannot tolerate the challenge of questioning; nurses by title only who are removed from direct patient care; or poorly educated nurse's aides, charged with the intimate bedside care of patients. We no longer see the untutored technologist who was ignorant of how to meet the needs of frightened, anxious patients; the hospital administrator who never visited patients at bedside; and the board of trustees whose members were isolated from and unexposed to the daily needs of patients. We no longer face negative societal and political attitudes and negative financial balances in hospitals and the health care community.

What we learned from the past has led to improvements: expansion of home care; visitation by social service, nurses, and physicians; direct communication for the patient from the continuing care support center; financial support of the patient; psychosocial support of the family or friends of the patient; and easy road transportation to and from the support center available for all patients.

The physical design and operation of the support center were carried over from St. Christopher's Hospice. There are special consideration and recognition by the clinical staff when the patient comes into the emergency room. The patient is not a stranger. He always receives information about the center at the door so that he feels comfortable in it and can meet its bureaucracy—the doctor, the nurse, the technicians, and everyone else.

Patients are considered as adults, even if they have regressed. (A psychiatrist would say that we all regress.) We do not treat our patients as children; we face their anxieties and frights and make them feel in control.

We have reconstituted the familiar personal environment that existed in St. Christopher's. We remember what a physician was like when a patient refused treatment. Now we avoid negative carryover to nurses, house staff, and technicians when the patient does refuse. We respect the patient's right to refuse blood drawing, especially by the incompetent and untrained.

We listen to the patient who has special knowledge of his own idiosyncratic reactions to certain treatments. The physician now assures the patient and provides the means whereby he or she can be called directly by the patient. We do not use the nurse or the answering service as a barrier; neither do we isolate a community of patients in private or semiprivate rooms.

We were always after the patient—he was wrong; he did not do as we ordered; he was a terrible person! The physician's responsibility has been reassessed. The physician must be available and must explain what will happen to the patient in the center. The physician explains the personality quirks of an individual patient to nurses and house staff and does not reinforce staff's negative attitudes; the physician has a willingness to be *used* by the patient within broad boundaries. Nurses have rethought their training, and there are more clinical nurses. Perhaps they are paid the same amount as doctors because they do take care of the patients.

The center has a religious base; without it (whether or not one is a believer) no hospice or continuing care service can go on. We used to forget about recreation, but now we have it in our budgets.

All of these innovations confront the regression of individuals who are hospitalized and chronically ill. The objective is to handle the patient's frustrations, loneliness, and depression. We use group interaction so that people draw strength and enrichment from one another. We support emotional education; we pay attention to the family, children, spouses, and close friends who may be the only family. We help the staff resolve and prevent despair. We provide a community for hope and life.

Index

Contributors

AUSTIN H. KUTSCHER, President, The Foundation of Thanatology; Professor of Dentistry (in Psychiatry), Department of Psychiatry, College of Physicians and Surgeons, Columbia University; Professor of Dentistry (in Psychiatry), School of Dental and Oral Surgery, Columbia University, New York, New York

SAMUEL C. KLAGSBRUN, M.D., Associate Clinical Professor, Department of Psychiatry, College of Physicians and Surgeons, Columbia University, New York, New York; Medical Director, Four Winds Hospital, Katonah, New York

RICHARD J. TORPIE, M.D., Department of Radiation Therapy, St. Luke's Hospital, Bethlehem, Pennsylvania

ROBERT DeBELLIS, M.D., Assistant Professor of Clinical Medicine, College of Physicians and Surgeons, Columbia University, New York, New York

MAHLON S. HALE, M.D., Associate Professor of Psychiatry and Director of Psychiatric Consultation Service, University of Connecticut Health Sciences Center, Farmington, Connecticut

MARGOT TALLMER, Ph.D., Professor of Psychology, Hunter College of the City University of New York, New York

RUTH D. ABRAMS, M.S., A.C.S.W., Private Practice, Cambridge, Massachusetts; Author

JAMES G. ANDERSON, Ph.D., Professor of Sociology, Department of Sociology and Anthropology, Purdue University, West Lafayette, Indiana; Division of Academic Affairs, Methodist Hospital of Indiana, Inc., Indianapolis, Indiana

JOAN E. ANDERSON, M.A., Professor of Applied Ethics, College for Human Service, New York, New York; Adjunct Professor, Bergen County Community College, New Jersey

HYLAN A. BICKERMAN, M.D., Clinical Professor of Medicine, College of Physicians and Surgeons, Columbia University, New York, New York

MARTIN BLACKSTEIN, Ph.D., M.D., Associate Professor of Medicine and Anatomy (Histology), University of Toronto; Director of Oncology, Mt. Sinai Hospital, Toronto, Ontario, Canada

ROBERT W. BUCKINGHAM, Dr. P.H., Associate Professor, Family and Community Medicine, University of Arizona, Tucson, Arizona

ARTHUR C. CARR, Ph.D., Professor of Clinical Psychology in Psychiatry, Cornell University Medical College, New York Hospital—Westchester Division, White Plains, New York

LO-YI CHAN, F.A.I.A., Partner, Prentice and Chan, Ohlhausen, Architects and Planners, New York, New York

JAMES E. CIMINO, M.D., Clinical Professor of Medicine, New York Medical College; Attending Physician, Calvary Hospital, Bronx, New York; formerly, Medical Director, Calvary Hospital, Bronx, New York

ELIZABETH J. COLERICK, R.N., M.S., Doctoral Candidate, Cornell University, Ithaca, New York

ALFONS DEEKEN, Ph.D., Professor of Philosophy, Sophia University, Tokyo, Japan

ROBERTA FILICKY-PENESKI, Community Programs Consultant, Sheboygan, Wisconsin

WILLIAM F. FINN, M.D., Associate Professor of Obstetrics and Gynecology, Cornell University Medical College, New York, New York; Attending Gynecologist, North Shore University Hospital, Manhasset, New York

PAMELA GRAY-TOFT, Ph.D., Vice President of Human Resources and Organization Development, Methodist Hospital of Indiana, Inc., Indianapolis, Indiana

JOHN E. HARE, Ph.D., Associate Professor, Department of Philosophy, Lehigh University, Bethlehem, Pennsylvania

AUDREY G. HARRIS, M.P.H., M.S.W., C.S.W., Senior Health Planner, Comprehensive Planning Council of Southeastern Michigan, Detroit, Michigan

RUSSELL JAFFE, Ph.D., M.D., formerly, United States Public Health Service, Bethesda, Maryland

LILLIAN G. KUTSCHER, Publications Editor, The Foundation of Thanatology, New York, New York

LEONARD M. LIEGNER, M.D., Associate Clinical Professor of Radiology, College of Physicians and Surgeons, Columbia University; Director, Radiation Therapy, St. Luke's-Roosevelt Hospital Center, New York, New York

WILLIAM LISS-LEVINSON, Ph.D., Director, The Brooklyn Hospice at Metropolitan Jewish Geriatric Center, Brooklyn, New York

DONALD MALAFRONTE, Director, Urban Health Institute, Roseland, New Jersey

ELLEN MARTIN, M.A., Director of Patient Relations, St. Luke's-Roosevelt Hospital Center, New York, New York

LUIS F. MARTORELL, M.S.W., A.C.S.W., B.C.S.W., Assistant Professor, Tulane University School of Social Work, New Orleans, Louisiana

SHARON McMAHON, R.N., Toronto, Ontario, Canada

RICHARD A. METZ, M.H.A., Administrator, Division of Transplantation, University of Miami School of Medicine, Miami, Florida

DAVID W. MOLLER, Ph.D., Assistant Professor, Department of Sociology, Fort Hays State University, Fort Hays, Kansas

RABBI STEVEN A. MOSS, Senior Chaplain, Memorial Sloan-Kettering Cancer Center, New York, New York; Spiritual Leader, B'nai Israel Reform Temple, Oakdale, New York

DEAN B. PRATT, M.D., F.A.C.S., Sheboygan Clinic, Sheboygan, Wisconsin

JOSEPH R. PROULX, R.N., Ed.D., Professor of Nursing, University of Maryland School of Nursing, Baltimore, Maryland

WILLIAM REGELSON, M.D., Professor of Medicine, Virginia Commonwealth University, Medical College of Virginia, Richmond, Virginia

MARY ROMANO, C.S.W., Assistant Director, Department of Social Work Services, The Presbyterian Hospital in the City of New York, New York

ARLENE SEGUINE, Ed.D., Associate Professor of Gerontology/Thanatology, Department of Health and Physical Education, Hunter College of the City University of New York, New York

VIRGINIA MONTERO SEPLOWIN, D.S.W., Director, Right Human Relations Center, New York, New York

EGILDE SERAVALLI, Ph.D., Department of Anesthesiology, Beth Israel Hospital and Medical Center, New York, New York

FLORENCE S. WALD, R.N., M.S., F.A.A.N., Yale University Graduate School of Nursing, New Haven, Connecticut

HENRY J. WALD, P.E., Consulting Engineer, Jansen and Rogan, New Haven, Connecticut

ELEANOR WASSERMAN, R.N., Coordinator of Oncology, Mt. Sinai Hospital, Toronto, Ontario, Canada

BRIAN WEST, Ph.D., Assistant Professor of Psychology, Medical University of South Carolina, College of Medicine, Charleston, South Carolina

PETER G. WILSON, M.D., Associate Professor of Psychiatry, Cornell University Medical Center, New York, New York

Columbia University Press/Foundation of Thanatology Series

Teaching Psychosocial Aspects of Patient Care
Bernard Schoenberg, Helen F. Pettit, and Arthur C. Carr, editors

Loss and Grief: Psychological Management in Medical Practice
Bernard Schoenberg, Arthur C. Carr, David Peretz, and Austin H. Kutscher, editors

Psychosocial Aspects of Terminal Care
Bernard Schoenberg, Arthur C. Carr, David Peretz, and Austin H. Kutscher, editors

Psychosocial Aspects of Cystic Fibrosis: A Model for Chronic Lung Disease
Paul R. Patterson, Carolyn R. Denning, and Austin H. Kutscher, editors

The Terminal Patient: Oral Care
Austin H. Kutscher, Bernard Schoenberg, and Arthur C. Carr, editors

Psychopharmacologic Agents for the Terminally Ill and Bereaved
Ivan K. Goldberg, Sidney Malitz, and Austin H. Kutscher, editors

Anticipatory Grief
Bernard Schoenberg, Arthur C. Carr, Austin H. Kutscher, David Peretz, and Ivan K. Goldberg, editors

Bereavement: Its Psychosocial Aspects
Bernard Schoenberg, Irwin Gerber, Alfred Wiener, Austin H. Kutscher, David Peretz, and Arthur C. Carr, editors

The Nurse as Caregiver for the Terminal Patient and His Family
Ann M. Earle, Nina T. Argondizzo, and Austin H. Kutscher, editors

Social Work with the Dying Patient and the Family
Elizabeth R. Prichard, Jean Collard, Ben A. Orcutt, Austin H. Kutscher, Irene Seeland, and Nathan Lefkowitz, editors

Home Care: Living with Dying
Elizabeth R. Prichard, Jean Collard, Janet Starr, Josephine A. Lockwood, Austin H. Kutscher, and Irene B. Seeland, editors

Psychosocial Aspects of Cardiovascular Disease: The Life-Threatened Patient, the Family, and the Staff.
James Reiffel, Robert DeBellis, Lester C. Mark, Austin H. Kutscher, Paul R. Patterson, and Bernard Schoenberg, editors

Acute Grief: Counseling the Bereaved
Otto S. Margolis, Howard C. Raether, Austin H. Kutscher, J. Bruce Powers, Irene B. Seeland, Robert DeBellis, and Daniel J. Cherico, editors

The Human Side of Homicide
Bruce L. Danto, John Bruhns, and Austin H. Kutscher, editors

Hospice U.S.A.
Austin H. Kutscher, Samuel C. Klagsbrun, Richard J. Torpie, Robert DeBellis, Mahlon S. Hale, and Margot Tallmer, editors

The Child and Death
John E. Schowalter, Paul R. Patterson, Margot Tallmer, Austin H. Kutscher, Stephen V. Gullo, and David Peretz, editors

HOSPICE U.S.A.

**Austin H. Kutscher, Samuel C. Klagsbrun,
Richard J. Torpie, Robert DeBellis,
Mahlon S. Hale, Margot Tallmer, Editors**

With the editorial assistance of
Lillian G. Kutscher

Continuing the Foundation of Thanatology series, *Hospice U.S.A.* introduces the hospice—its history, philosophy, and current status in the United States. The hospice movement, as it is now conceptualized, originated in England in the late 1950s as a facility where terminally ill patients could receive appropriate care in an atmosphere designed to ease the stresses of physical and emotional suffering. From its start, this kind of caregiving has advanced itself internationally and now is being practiced or planned in almost 1000 locales in this country.

According to the editors, "present-day hospice means an attitude, a concept, a service. As a service it may take place in an institution exclusively devoted to it or may be practiced in alternative sites. It may be part of a hospital service, in a separate unit, or as an interdisciplinary program covering terminally ill patients assigned to rooms throughout the building. It may include a home care program providing round-the-clock team service, an outpatient or daycare program, or be sponsored by one institution or in cooperation with many others. Whatever its form, its ultimate goal is the same: to respect the dying and allow them to end their days in harmony."

Hospice U.S.A. consists of thirty-six essays collected under the headings "The Hospice Movement: Past and Present," "Ethical and Human Issues in Terminal Care," "Hospice Caregiving," "Helping the Dying: Caregiver Approaches," "Patients and Illnesses," "Alternatives to In-Hospice Care," and "A Look to the Future." In